Promoting Health and Well-being in Social Work Education

T0264740

Social work educators can play an important part in ensuring that the promotion of health and well-being is firmly on the social work agenda for service users, as well as for students and educators. Nevertheless, this has not been a priority within social work education and presents a challenge which requires some re-thinking in terms of curriculum content, pedagogy, and how social workers respond to social problems. Furthermore, if the promotion of health and well-being is not considered a priority for social workers, this raises important questions about the role and relevance of social work in health, and thus poses challenges to social work education, both now and in the future.

This book contains contributions from social work educators from Australia, Canada, New Zealand, the UK and the USA. They reflect on how best to prepare students to put health and well-being to the forefront of practice, drawing on research on quality of life, subjective well-being, student well-being, community participation and social connectedness, religion and spirituality, mindful practices, trauma and health inequalities.

This book is an extended version of a special issue of *Social Work Education*.

Beth R. Crisp is Professor in the School of Health and Social Development at Deakin University, Australia. Her teaching and research interests include addressing poverty and social exclusion, the relationship between religion and spirituality with social work practice, and workforce development.

Liz Beddoe is Professor in the School of Counselling, Human Services and Social Work at the University of Auckland, New Zealand. Her teaching and research interests include critical perspectives on social work education, professional supervision, the professionalization project of social work, interprofessional learning and the development of health social work.

Promoting Health and Well-being in Social Work Education

Edited by
Beth R. Crisp and Liz Beddoe

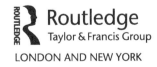

Routledge
Taylor & Francis Group

LONDON AND NEW YORK

First published 2013
by Routledge
2 Park Square, Milton Park, Abingdon, Oxfordshire OX14 4RN

Simultaneously published in the USA and Canada
by Routledge
711 Third Avenue, New York, NY 10017

First issued in paperback 2014

Routledge is an imprint of the Taylor & Francis Group, an informa business

This book is an extended version of *Social Work Education*, volume 30, issue 6. The Publisher requests to those authors who may be citing this book to state, also, the bibliographical details of the special issue in which each article was originally published.

Trademark notice: Product or corporate names may be trademarks or registered trademarks, and are used only for identification and explanation without intent to infringe.

British Library Cataloguing in Publication Data
A catalogue record for this book is available from the British Library

ISBN 978-0-415-52798-9 (hbk)
ISBN 978-1-138-84186-4 (pbk)

Typeset in Sabon LT Std and Gill Sans Std
by Saxon Graphics Ltd, Derby

Publisher's Note
The publisher would like to make readers aware that most of the chapters in this book may be referred to as articles as they are identical to the articles previously published in the journal *Social Work Education*. The publisher accepts responsibility for any inconsistencies that may have arisen in the course of preparing this volume for print.

Contents

CONTENTS

Citation Information

The following chapters were originally published in the journal *Social Work Education*. When citing this material, please use the original issue information and page numbering for each article, as follows:

Chapter 3
   The contribution of social work and social interventions across the life course to the reduction of health inequalities: A new agenda for social work education?
   Esther Coren, Wendy Iredale, Deborah Rutter and Paul Bywaters
   Social Work Education, volume 30, issue 6 (September 2011) pp. 594–609

Chapter 4
   Health and Wellbeing: Starting with a Critical Pedagogical Model
   Rachelle Ashcroft
   Social Work Education, volume 30, issue 6 (September 2011) pp. 610–622

Chapter 5
   Teaching trauma: Critically engaging with a troublesome term
   Jay Marlow and Carole Adamson
   Social Work Education, volume 30, issue 6 (September 2011) pp. 623–634

Chapter 6
   Developing wellbeing as a critical tool in social work education: An example from the field of learning disability
   Graeme Simpson
   Social Work Education, volume 31, issue 5 (August 2012) pp. 622–636

Chapter 7
   From theory toward empathic self-care: Creating a mindful classroom for social work students
   Maria Napoli and Robin Bonifas
   Social Work Education, volume 30, issue 6 (September 2011) pp. 635–649

Notes on Contributors

Carole Adamson, University of Auckland, NZ

Rachelle Ashcroft, Wilfrid Laurier University, Canada

Liz Beddoe, University of Auckland, NZ

Robin Bonifas, Arizona State University, USA

Paul Bywaters, Coventry University, UK

Esther Coren, Canterbury Christ Church University, UK

Beth R. Crisp, Deakin University, Australia

Christa Fouché, University of Auckland, NZ

Mel Hughes, University of Bournemouth, UK

Wendy Iredale, Sheffield Hallam University, UK

Selma Macfarlane, Deakin University, Australia

Jane Maidment, Christchurch Polytechnic Institute of Technology, NZ

Jay Marlow, University of Auckland, NZ

Kathy Martindale, University of Auckland, NZ

Jo Mensinga, James Cook University, Australia

Maria Napoli, Arizona State University, USA

Deborah Rutter, Social Care Institute for Excellence, UK

Graeme Simpson, University of Wolverhampton, UK

Introduction: Promoting Health and Well-Being in Social Work Education

Beth R. Crisp and Liz Beddoe

It is now 25 years since the influential Ottawa Charter for Health Promotion clearly outlined an agenda which positioned health as a valuable resource, and recognised the contribution of not just the health sector in promoting health and well-being:

> Health promotion is the process of enabling people to increase control over, and to improve, their health. To reach a state of complete physical, mental and social wellbeing, an individual or group must be able to identify and to realize aspirations, to satisfy needs, and to change or cope with the environment. Health is, therefore, seen as a resource for everyday life, not the objective of living. Health is a positive concept emphasizing social and personal resources, as well as physical capacities. Therefore, health promotion is not just the responsibility of the health sector, but goes beyond healthy life-styles to well-being. (World Health Organization, 1986)

More recently, the International Federation of Social Workers in its 2008 policy statement 'International Policy on Health' (IFSW, 2008) has described health as an issue of fundamental importance for social work practice. The IFSW argues that the promotion of health and well-being is aligned with the core social work values of human rights and social justice. While access to appropriate health services should be a right, too many people in the world cannot take this for granted, including many in our own countries which are among the world's richest nations. As long as social workers must continue to work to ensure that individuals and communities have adequate resources such as education, food, housing, clothing as well as the financial and social support necessary to thrive and develop to one's full potential, social workers will necessarily be involved in health issues (Bywaters, McLeod & Napier, 2009). As the IFSW statement notes, 'Social workers in all settings are engaged in health work whether in creating the conditions for improved health chances or working alongside people to manage the impact of poor health on themselves or those close to them' (IFSW, 2008).

It is not just in service provision, but also in policy development, where the IFSW sees an important role for social workers in promoting health and well-being. Unfortunately, social workers have too often been active in promoting programmes and policies which have actually had a deleterious effect on health and well-being of individuals and communities. Hence in its recommendations about the roles and responsibilities of social workers, the IFSW has recommended that:

> All social workers should constantly question the health consequences of their actions. IFSW policy opposes overt or covert actions or policies which are discriminatory or which exacerbate health inequalities. For example, policies and practices involving indigenous peoples and child migrants have sometimes resulted in the destruction of family and community life and life long physical and emotional health problems. Social workers should pay attention to the economic and political roots of the troubles people bring to them and give sufficient attention to ensuring that service recipients have a say in the direction and priorities of service provision. (IFSW, 2008)

The IFSW perspective on the social work role in the promotion of health and well-being is not universally understood within the profession. Certainly the promotion of health and well-being has long been (going back to a period even earlier than the Ottawa Charter) considered a significant and legitimate objective of social work practice in some parts of the world. In the 21st century there is wide variation in social work participation in health care services and programmes. In many countries health social work is a significant field of practice located mainly in institutional (private and government) hospitals and community services. Social workers are also employed in the fields of public health and health promotion in policy, planning and research as well as in direct practice in primary health care and in 'grassroots' advocacy and support organisations. Broad and holistic approaches to well-being provide a significant focus for working with vulnerable groups, especially in the fields of mental health, disability and services to support older adults.

We are nevertheless aware that for many social workers the promotion of health and well-being is not a key consideration, either for themselves or for the agencies in which they are employed. As social workers in Australia and New Zealand, where there has long been social work involvement in health services and health promotion, during the preparation of this volume we have been surprised by the number of encounters we have had with prospective authors who have suggested that this is a new agenda for the social work profession. However, given the prominence in recent years, at least in the professional literature, on risk management and ameliorating individual deficits, the potential for social work to impact more broadly on well-being can readily be lost. Fawcett (2009, p. 474) notes that the emphasis on risk assessment and safety focussed interventions while well-meaning can lead to disempowerment through a failure 'to place the individual at the heart of the decision to intervene and which fail to engage adequately with their experiences'. Social work thus has a role to play in critically assessing policies that overly focus on functional incapacity and associated vulnerabilities rather than personal aspirations, potential and social connectedness.

As the chapters in this volume demonstrate, social work educators can play an important contribution in ensuring that promoting health and well-being are firmly on the social work agenda for service users as well as for our students and ourselves as educators. Nevertheless, we recognise that this may be a challenge which requires some re-thinking in terms of curriculum content, pedagogy, and the theoretical standpoints that influence how social workers respond to social problems (Bacchi, 2009). However, if the promotion of health and well-being is not considered a priority for social workers, this raises important questions about the role and relevance of social work, and hence social work education, both now and in the future. In the following chapter, Beddoe describes what has too often been a problematic status quo of social work education tending to ignore or provide minimal coverage of health in the curriculum or relegate it to a minor subject status, usually an elective. Health is also often conceptualized within social work education in a very limited manner as being about sickness and social work in hospitals. Health social work practice has historically been most prominent within institutional settings and as a consequence the knowledge identified as crucial in this field is influenced by the dominant biomedical paradigm. The location of social work in a host setting with its associated medical dominance often limits the acknowledgement of the social determinants of health and the potential to contribute to reduction of health disparities.

The remaining chapters within this volume reflect the breadth of scholarship and research that can be employed within social work education to best prepare students for a practice that puts health and well-being at the forefront of practice. Chapters from Australia, Canada, New Zealand, the United Kingdom and the United States of America provide a broad sweep of perspectives drawing on research on quality of life, subjective well-being, the impact of social work education on students' welfare, stress and trauma, community participation, religion and spirituality, mindful practices, disabilities and health inequalities.

Coren, Iredale, Rutter and Bywaters argue for a greater focus in social work education on the centrality of social aspects of physical and mental health in service users' lives. The chapter explores the potential for social work to contribute to the reduction of health inequalities within the framework provided by the UK General Social Care Council's *Codes of Practice for Social Care Workers* (2010). The examples provided offer an illustration of how awareness of health disparities can be woven into explorations of policy and practice. Ashcroft provides an overview of the six most dominant health paradigms: biomedicine, public health, biopsychosocial, social determinants of health, political economy, and holism. Understanding these varying perspectives and their compatibility with social work values provides tools for shaping practice in a way that best focuses on health and wellness. Marlowe and Adamson address the troublesome concept of trauma, which they find often utilised uncritically. Drawing on two research studies these authors illustrate that a social work construction of a trauma knowledge base can inform a vibrant and critical curriculum. Simpson then explores well-being in the field of learning disability by exploring three themes which have a much broader applicability than this single field of practice: friendships and relationships, community engagement, and structural factors.

From policies and paradigms, we turn to a much more practice-oriented focus. The focus broadens as a series of chapters consider the connections between mind, body, spirit and our intellectual and moral dimensions as apposite to the aims of social work education. Napoli and Bonifas describe the elements of a mindful classroom in social work education and utilising the results of a study that examined learning outcomes associated with mindfulness introduce a framework for teaching mindful practice. Mensinga draws both on the extensive literature of the mind–body connection and her own experience of using yoga as a reflexive practice to make the role of the body more visible in the professional discourse of social work. She argues that placing a greater emphasis on embodied knowledge in social work education will strengthen the reflexive capacity of graduates, support the health and well-being of social workers and as a consequence produce better outcomes for service users. Crisp considers the implications of developing curriculum which acknowledges the religious dimension of the lives of many service users, arguing that this is a neglected area in social work education. She suggests the need for skill development to enable social workers to broach issues of religion with service users; and develop their capacities for working in or with faith-based agencies. Fouché and Martindale propose that raising awareness of the core domains of life satisfaction during social work education will eventually enable more effective management of stress and burnout and quality of service delivery in practice through better work–life balance. Hughes explores the impact (positive and negative) of challenges to students' values and perspectives within social work education, drawing on a unitary appreciative inquiry. Hughes suggests further research is needed on the effectiveness of strategies for dealing with stress and stressful situations.

Maidment and Macfarlane address the significance to well-being of place and social space and the value of informal networks to generate support and opportunities for reciprocity. Drawing on a small research study of older women and craft making they explore how learning from diverse disciplines can illuminate understanding of well-being beyond a focus on illness and deterioration. In keeping with a significant theme of this special issue, the authors argue that by engaging with a more diverse range of disciplines, educators will be able to teach and advocate for well-being in more expansive and useful ways.

This collection of chapters highlights the knowledge base for understanding the impact of health, challenges to beliefs and values, work and academic stress and trauma in the lives of students, practitioners and service-users and the need to be aware of peoples' capacities to respond to difficult situations. In the concluding chapter we seek to draw out the key themes and issues which have been identified in this volume and make recommendations to support the promotion of health and well-being within social work education.

The majority of the chapters in this volume previously appeared in the special issue of *Social Work Education: The International Journal* (vol. 30, no. 6) published in October 2011. We wish to acknowledge the support of the journal's editors and editorial board, the majority of whom are based in the United Kingdom, for agreeing to support a special issue which emerged from our reflections on practice in Australia and New Zealand. We also wish to thank Routledge for the opportunity to expand the original special issue into this present volume. Finally, this volume would not have been possible without the contributions of all the authors who contributed to this project and in doing so vindicated our stance that the promotion of health and well-being is a crucial role for social work education.

References

Bacchi, C.L. (2009) *Analysing Policy: What's the Problem Represented to Be?* Pearson, Frenchs Forest, NSW.

Bywaters, P., McLeod, E. & Napier, L. (Eds.). (2009) *Social Work and Global Health Inequalities*, Policy Press, Bristol.

Fawcett, B. (2009). 'Vulnerability: Questioning the certainties in social work and health', *International Social Work*, vol. 52, no.4, pp. 473–484.

General Social Care Council (GSCC) (2010) *Codes of Practice for Social Care Workers*, GSCC, London.

International Federation of Social Workers (IFSW) (2008) *International Policy on Health*. Available at http://www.ifsw.org/en/p38000081.html, accessed 30 November 2011.

World Health Organization (WHO) (1986) The Ottawa Charter for Health Promotion [online]. Available at: http://www.who.int/healthpromotion/conferences/previous/ottawa/en/, accessed 1 May 2011.

Social Work Education and Health: Knowledge for Practice

Liz Beddoe

Health and well-being are often treated within social work education in a very limited manner as being about sickness and social work in hospitals. Health social work practice is most prominent within institutional settings in many countries and as a consequence the knowledge identified as crucial in this field is influenced by the dominant biomedical paradigm. Within the context of contemporary health services social work is commonly an auxiliary service within a 'host' organisation customarily organised around medical services. Social work must vie for space and resource for its unique perspective within this setting, while needing to 'fit in'. The knowledge base for practice is thus potentially full of competing and contested paradigms. This chapter explores these concerns and the implications for social work education. A wide-lens/ narrow-lens framework is suggested to foster inclusion of critical health perspectives throughout the curriculum.

Introduction

Health and well-being (or a lack thereof) is essential to our experiences of being human. We experience the world and our contributions to it from integration of our physical, emotional, spiritual, cognitive and cultural resources and limitations. As living to the best of our abilities is important to most people, the contribution of social factors to health and well-being should not be under-estimated. Health is not an equal commodity and social inequalities mean that within neighbourhoods, regions, countries, continents and oceans people start and finish in very different places in terms of their well-being (Keefe, 2010). A child in care who has missed essential checks in early childhood and has hearing difficulties has an early learning disadvantage that will interfere with his or her potential. Middle aged workers who have unsafe exposure to toxic materials may face lower quality of life in their older years. Being born into a specific population in an accident of geography may mean a child starts life with higher likelihood of becoming ill with particular diseases. Limited ability to control work and income means that some individuals experience more stress. Class and poverty may be seen as embodied within health status (Rose and Hatzenbuehler, 2009). These concerns are central to social work wherever it is practised. As such Bywaters and Napier write:

> Our view is that *social work is health work*. As we write in the [IFSW] policy, social workers in all settings engage every day with children, men and women struggling to realize their basic rights to health. It is not only social workers in health settings such as hospitals or clinics who must be concerned with health issues. (Bywaters and Napier, 2009, p. 453 [emphasis added])

If indeed we are all health workers, then health must be more visible in the profession. Social work education can make a more significant contribution to ensuring that the promotion of health and well-being is firmly on the agenda in our direct work with service users as well as for our students and ourselves as practitioners and professional educators. It is of concern that social work education tends to ignore or provide minimal coverage of health in the curriculum or relegate it to a minor subject status, usually an elective. There are very many competing priorities in designing curriculum for social work and countries differ in the extent to which their governments influence what is taught. Nevertheless, health has not been a priority within social work education (Bywaters and Napier, 2009) and presents a challenge requiring more exploration of both health-related curriculum content and pedagogy. Furthermore, if the advancement of health and well-being is not considered a priority in education this raises important questions about our profession's adherence to its statement of the fundamental centrality of health and well-being in social justice (International Federation of Social Workers [IFSW], 2008).

This chapter explores some of the opportunities for social work education to do more to promote an understanding of the significance of health while recognizing that this is not a straightforward undertaking. There are many potential approaches and what works will to large extent depend on the context of practice in each country. Bywaters, Cowden, McLeod, Rose and Singh (2009) suggest in their guidance in the Social Work and Policy Digest that there are three main ways to insert material related to health inequalities into the curriculum. The first method is 'permeation' where learning about health is spread throughout the teaching programme. A second approach is the development of specialist health modules or electives in programmes. A third suggested option is the development of interprofessional teaching to mixed groups of students in professional education programmes. The manner in which these opportunities to impart a 'health equality imagination' (Giles, 2009) impacts on the kind of social work we envisage. Coren, Iredale, Rutter and Bywaters (2011) suggest that social workers can contribute through many social interventions across the life course to the reduction of health inequalities and these perspectives need to be explored in curricula. The interaction of social workers with health and health services varies across the world. This chapter will address issues of context and explore the professional engagement of social workers within complex health systems. Implications for social work education are considered and a wide-lens/narrow-lens framework is suggested to foster inclusion of critical health perspectives throughout the curriculum.

Social Work in Health Care

The origins of the practice of social work in health care are found for the main part in host organisations. In its early days social work was promoted by other professions as an adjunct to public health services (Cabot, 1919; Todd, 1919). In many countries (for example Australia, New Zealand, Canada, Ireland, South Africa, the United States, Finland) social work in health services is a significant field of practice within the profession. In other countries social work in health may be more specialised (palliative care, mental health, user and advocacy organisations) and elsewhere the practice may be more closely linked to community development and public health. Social work in primary care offers the opportunity for practice closer to the 'front line' of health inequalities (McLeod, 2002). Primary care is essential health care; available in the community at an affordable cost and geared toward well-being and self-determination. In some countries there is considerable interest in developing social work in primary care—see for example work being done by the Irish Association of Social Workers [IASW] (2010); and in Canada by the Canadian Association of Social Workers (n.d.). In Ireland, for example, policy suggests primary care social workers are 'uniquely placed to engage in community development aspects of prevention and health promotion with the communities in which they work, through appropriate training and support from our community work colleagues' [IASW]. In the author's country, New Zealand, social work in primary care is in its infancy. Clearly there is a significant role for social work in primary health given the emphasis on primary care in public health strategies (see for example, Clark, 2011). The literature on health social work tends to reflect the domination of institutional practice in developed countries. Social work in health care has conventionally derived its professional identity from a claim to expertise in the 'psychosocial' aspects of illness, based on a longstanding perception that medical and nursing staff limited their focus on physical factors and treatment of service users in health systems (Roach-Anleu, 1992, pp. 40–41). As such the knowledge base for health practice has often reflected a focus on psychological and social functioning of those encountering the disruption of illness in personal and family life.

Contextualising this within a socioeconomic understanding of health and social disadvantage led Giles (2009, p. 526) to comment on her own practice in a busy hospital setting:

> I was experiencing immense pressure to work with the dominant individual biological and psychological understandings of health and to abandon principles of social and community responsibility for the well-being of others. This led me to deeply question the role of social work in health in a socio-political context dominated by ideas of conservatism and economic rationalism.

Giles (2009) points to the dominant discourses in health—biomedical, psychological—and the way these influence practice and suggests that social work is challenged by critical social theory to move our understanding of the social inequalities of health into sharper focus. Giles points to what may be the inadequacy of the biopsychosocial model for contemporary social work. Often narrowly interpreted, the 'social' component is often limited to the immediate circumstances of individuals and their families in contact with the health system—mainly concerned with their social supports and socioeconomic resources. Over the last decade there has been increasing emphasis on the need to highlight health inequalities in the curriculum for social work education (McLeod and Bywaters, 2002; Bywaters *et al.*, 2009; Giles, 2009; Keefe, 2010). At the same time awareness of the inequalities has been promoted through international advocacy with the development of the IFSW policy statement on health (IFSW, 2008). The Social Work and Health Inequalities Network, an international network of social workers, was formed in 2004 with 'aims to promote research, discussion and action by social work researchers, educators, practitioners and managers, to combat the causes and consequences of unjust and damaging socially created inequalities in health' (n.p).

Knowledge and Social Work Identity

How then do we ensure that social workers are well informed about health, inclusive of health disparities, regardless of the field of practice they enter on graduation? Decisions made about curriculum are not innocent; they reflect the tensions and competing discourses within the profession and in the wider society. The knowledge base for the profession is significant beyond day to day considerations of time, resources and expertise. Elsewhere I have explored the professionalization of social work through the particular lens of professional capital (Beddoe, 2010; 2011a) where knowledge and identity are inescapably linked. Professional capital comprises many significant attributes and of particular significance for social work in health are the following key elements: members of the profession are able to 'make a clear and understood knowledge-claim for practice ... including both the application and production of knowledge; a clear and well differentiated territory of practice, ... and the particular profession is visible in the public discourse of the contributions professions make to society and is particular and recognizable for its distinctive contribution to social well-being' (Beddoe, 2010, pp. 10–16). Olgiati notes that in defining a profession, a 'common pattern ... is the connection of profession with a particular educational preparation and the practice of a particular type of knowledge, basically academic knowledge' (Olgiati, 2006, pp. 540–541), often termed the 'knowledge claim'. The social work profession has often overruled the making of an outright knowledge claim as elitist (Green, 2006), while at the same time trusting that our distinctive approach will be recognised and respected, especially in complex organisational contexts.

Social work has however sought some degree of occupational closure, wishing to have some ability to protect vulnerable groups of service users from the impact of poor practice (Dominelli, 1996). The impact of the risk society (Beck, 1992) on the social work profession (Webb, 2006) and the associated rise of powerful public scrutiny have also led governments to legislate for registration of practitioners, where self-regulation was deemed inadequate (Orme and Rennie, 2006). A focus on 'at risk' and vulnerable communities in society is notable in contemporary health care, as universal tools such as family violence screening become part of the everyday practice. Healy (2009) has observed that within the current 'new public management' regime, professions who can prove 'their capacity to manage risk through reference to a scientific evidence base', hold credibility while those who employ 'interpretivist or critical approaches to knowledge development ... are vulnerable to devaluation' (p. 402). This is of particular significance to social workers in traditional health settings where social work activity is framed by expectations of the host organisation (Roach-Anleu, 1992; Giles *et al.*, 2007).

In health settings social workers seek to secure greater professional capital, often seeing their role as importantly challenging biomedical dominance within institutional settings while in reality there may only be an uneasy coexistence (Beddoe, 2011a). For social work there is a constant challenge to achieve improved visibility in the public discourse and greater recognition of the profession's distinctive contribution to social well-being. There is broad agreement in the literature about the role of social work in health and the inherent challenges practitioners face in almost universally financially constrained, stretched and struggling health services (Giles *et al.*, 2007). The desire to be seen as adding value underpins much contemporary focus in the development of the profession in health (Nilsson, Ryan and Miller, 2007; Auerbach, Mason and Heft La Porte, 2007; Auerbach and Mason, 2010). The role of research activity, including utilisation is the focus of much discussion as well, often with an emphasis on raising the standing of the profession and its contribution to knowledge (Joubert, 2006; Björkenheim, 2007; Beddoe, 2011b).

The wider health context drives some of this new enthusiasm for linking knowledge to the identity and standing of the profession, especially for social workers in health (Beddoe, 2011a; 2011b). The development of evidence-based practice (EBP) challenges the potency of an exclusive knowledge claim for any profession. While many social workers might view EBP as symbolic of medical dominance, some deconstruction of this suggests it represents a weakening of power. EBP aims to evaluate practices against other practices, using so-called gold standard methods. The result of these projects creates codified knowledge packaged as 'Best Practice'. Through technologies of control such as 'clinical governance', bureaucracies assert control of professions. Social work involvement in health services are generally mediated via third parties in host organisations and social work independence is generally 'restricted by a tenacious, nervous managerialism that resists professional autonomy' (Beddoe, 2010, p. 256).

Health in the Social Work Curriculum

In the current environment health social work frames its professional values, aspirations and challenges within the constraints and opportunities within the structural arrangements of the host institutions. With renewed focus and a wider vision, social work education can thus assist the potential re-definition and strengthening of a social work practice in which a far-reaching commitment to enhancing well-being is central. Following on from Bywaters *et al.*'s identification of both permeation and specialist inputs (2009) it is proposed here that a two- pronged approach be taken to consideration of the 'health' curriculum for social work. The theoretical perspectives commonly utilized in main curriculum for social work include the following: critical social theory; ecological theory, family systems theory, understandings of human resiliency; social psychology; the study of the life course and the psychosocial impact of loss, trauma and grief. Common frameworks of knowledge for health include: a biopsychosocial model of health and the social models of health and disability. Aiming to extend these models, Cameron and McDermott (2007) developed a 'camera' approach—recognising the need for social workers to incorporate a wide view along with 'middle-distance' and 'close-up view' of health and well-being. It is suggested here that a similar framework can be developed for the curriculum to ensure health awareness and the contributions of critical perspectives are promoted within social work education. This framework includes two perspectives, a 'wide-lens view' and 'narrow-lens' view of curriculum depicted in Figures 1 and 2 respectively. Each can contribute to a good understanding of health and well-being, drawing on different perspectives. As Ashcroft (2011) points out perspectives such as biomedical, biopsychosocial, holistic and others all have particular epistemological underpinnings but in this chapter space precludes exploration of these in depth. Nor does this chapter purport to be an all-inclusive set of 'topics' for the curriculum relating to health and well-being. Mind–body connections, subjective well-being and work–life balance for example are important but are addressed by other contributors to this volume. Rather the wide- and narrow-lens framework is offered here to illustrate simply how social and critical perspectives of health understanding can be explored throughout a social work degree, not just within specialist content.

A broad view of health for social work practice: A wide-lens curriculum

This framework suggests that all social work students are exposed to information about the social inequalities of health and the impact of environment on the potential of individuals and communities. The shift to incorporate a wide-lens approach to health and its significance for social work is supported by the IFSW Policy Statement on Health (IFSW, 2008). The recognition of health as a social good and as such subject to inequalities had been promoted since the 1980s. In 1986 the highly significant Ottawa Charter for Health Promotion positioned health as a valuable human and social resource, and taking a wide view of human well-being, recognised the contribution of more than just the institutional health sector in promoting health and well-being:

> To reach a state of complete physical, mental and social well-being, an individual or group must be able to identify and to realize aspirations, to satisfy needs, and to change or cope with the environment. Health is, therefore, seen as a resource for everyday life, not the objective of living. Health is a positive concept emphasizing social and personal resources, as well as physical capacities. (World Health Organization, 1986)

Five action areas for health promotion were identified in the charter: building healthy public policy; creating supportive environments; strengthening community action; developing personal skills and lastly re-orientating health care services toward prevention of illness and promotion of health. Contributing to a broad public health agenda is a valid objective for social work practice, however the contribution of social work profession in response to the Ottawa aspirations is quite variable. In the Australian context Whiteside notes there is room and potential for partnerships in addressing the social determinants of health, despite 'historical differences in these two fields, with public health focusing on population level change and social work's interest lying primarily with individuals and communities' (2004, pp. 381–382). Many efforts have been made to combine social work and aspects of health promotion and public health in the United States; for example in describing a joint education programme, Ruth et al. (2008, p. 72) assert that 'social work and public health share a social justice mission to improve, defend, and enhance well-being, working together to ameliorate social health problems'. Social workers now may be found employed in the fields of population health and health promotion in policy, planning and research as well as in direct practice in primary health care and in advocacy organisations. Such dispersal of social work beyond traditional sites of delivery may be seen as shifting more towards population-based approaches, closer to the communities served (Vourlekis, Ell and Padgett, 2001).

Presenting students with an ecological approach to social work and health promotes a message that health and well-being are influenced by features of the physical, social, political and cultural environment. Holistic approaches to health alongside an awareness of the social determinants of poor health outcomes both provide a particularly effective focus for working with vulnerable groups. Critical reflection on the nature of human agency within the complex social and physical environment is pertinent. There are two static positions at either end of a spectrum of human agency; one being that lifestyle, behaviour, diet and culture are choices exercised in the way individuals and families conduct their lives; the other that many of these health choices are really 'factors'—features of a predetermined social structure in which a person has little or no choice. If one subscribes to this latter viewpoint then people are born into geographical, physical, social, cultural and environmental conditions over which they have very little choice. Illness, accident or the impact of natural disasters will be viewed as a disruption to normal expectations of life for individuals, families and communities. In the former view, health may be seen as signified by the absence of disease or causative factors and thus seen as within human control to some extent. Taking a fixed position on either view is unrealistic; individuals, families and communities can make choices, but their options are restricted by the unequal distribution of resources. A social habitat may include poor housing, the lack of amenities, weak social planning, limited resources for recreation and culture, and environmental damage.

Extensive research in many countries on social determinants of health has led to the development of many different kinds of interventions to address health inequalities (Bywaters *et al.*, 2009). Whitehead (2007, p. 474) categorised the types of interventions: strengthening individuals; strengthening communities; improving living and working conditions and promoting healthy macro-policies. The conceptual framework and research base of the social determinants of health approach can contribute to curriculum throughout social work education, especially when considering the human life course and the causes of family violence and neglect. When an impoverished environment forms the starting point in a life course, family and interpersonal violence, racism and sexism, ableism, barriers for people with disabilities and other forms of oppression have a greater corrosive impact. The WHO Commission on the Social Determinants of Health (2008) notes that the more adverse the social circumstance for individuals and in communities, the greater the impact of these factors on health outcomes. Greater attention to child neglect and the human life course is underscored by research on the impact of the whole environment. Whitehead (2007) notes that a life course approach is often applied, in recognition that 'a poor start in life, for example, severely limits children's opportunities to achieve their full health potential throughout life' (p. 476). Littrell (2008, p. 19) notes that 'childhood poverty and adversities experienced during childhood have been shown to have consequences for immune system function in adulthood. This, in turn, underscores the imperative of creating a more just society in which the gap between the rich and the poor is minimized'. Coren *et al.* (2010) in an excellent review of research have provided case studies of how social programmes can attack health disparities. Such a review can provide rich material for deepening social workers' understanding of health.

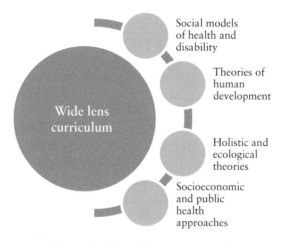

Figure 1 The wide lens curriculum

Introduction to social models of disability is part of the wide approach. A social model defines disability as 'the disadvantage or restriction of activity caused by a contemporary social organisation which takes little or no account of people who have physical impairments and thus excludes them from participation in the mainstream of social activities' (Union of the Physically Impaired Against Segregation and the Disability Alliance, 1976, np). The development of affirmative approaches to disability is an excellent case study for consideration in teaching social policy. Stigma, unnecessary social and financial barriers and disabling physical environments all impact on human potential and contribute to health disparities. There is a strong critical approach of contemporary significance, for despite significant improvement in the development of 'client-defined needs, desires and choices', Meekosha and Dowse point out that

> Service delivery organisations are still heavily involved with regulating and
> conditioning disabled people to accept responsibility for minimising their own

difference. Such regimes pursue a model of the rational, competent and independent citizenship, thus echoing the 'adjust' and 'adapt' mentality of earlier approaches. (Meekosha and Dowse, 2007, p. 172)

Discussion of the way in which 'the risk society' (Beck, 1992) has influenced the delivery of health and social services is relevant to social policy as well as social work practice. Vojak (2009) argues that neoliberal discourse has communicated concerns about 'efficiency and accountability, while dulling the concern for real people by objectifying and quantifying their lives' (p. 939). For example, risk-averse organisational cultures prioritise dealing with risk through many tools and technologies. In doing so Vojak argues that 'caring about community members who need assistance is not a primary motivating factor; keeping them from interfering with the lives and economic interests of others is' (p. 939). Thus people with complex needs and concerns who require care services are categorised distinctly as different from the rest of the community: 'Risk management language fails to appreciate how individual and community interests are overlapping and interwoven; it therefore neglects the bigger picture, ignoring possible long-term, systemic and preventative solutions' (p. 939). There is little focus in such policy on community strengths and personal and family resilience. Case studies including service users with chronic health concerns, disabilities and frail older adults can be used to illustrate the influence of risk-averse policy, rather than the more typical child protection focus.

'Place' becomes more significant when considering the impact of features of both the built and natural environment. A deeper discussion of the meaning of the environment within the traditional 'person-in-environment' schema must inevitably address geography and climate. Recently the links between the physical environment and social work have been cited as requiring attention (Besthorn, 2003; Kemp, 2011; McKinnon, 2008). McKinnon (2008, p. 257) argues that a debate on the response of the profession to the environmental crisis might go to the 'very heart of the way social work, as a profession, is defined and the boundaries of its professional domain'. Zapf (2008) argues that social work has recognised the importance of the natural and physical environment as exemplified in the phrase 'person-in-environment'. However in practice Zapf (2008, p. 175) argues the natural environment is invariably 'dropped from view' and transformed into the social environment. The degradation of the earth's resources of air, water, soil, and atmosphere and the negative impact on human well-being of this damage suggests that social workers must learn about environmental problems, and attendant oppressions (Coates, 2003). Zapf (2008) claims that international social work and sustainable development also offers advanced conceptualisations of the relationship between natural environment and human life that social workers could incorporate into the core of the profession.

Specific content for social work in health care: Narrowing the lens?

Narrowing the lens however does not mean focusing on micro processes of practice; the integration of wide and narrow lens approaches into the practice curriculum should be self-evident. Rather here I want to explore how material drawn from social sciences can be harnessed to deepen our understanding of how individuals and their loved ones experience health and illness, in the close-up view of everyday practice. This starts from an assumption that the sociology of health and illness is often very marginally visible in social work curriculum. Mainstream teaching and textbooks have tended towards the psychological discourse including narrow conceptualizations of resilience. A sociological approach enables us to imagine and think beyond our own experience of phenomena and challenge overly reductionist approaches to health and well-being. Challenges to the mind–body dualism have influenced contemporary health care and social workers certainly do not have exclusive claims to 'the social' in health and well-being.

An interesting and challenging topic for inclusion in social work education for health practice (though ideally given room elsewhere in the curricula as well) is that of social work and the body. Citing Turner (1992), Elliott discusses how social science had separated the self from the body. In mainstream sociology the body was often 'seen as a biological constraint upon human agency and social action' (Elliott, 2009, p. 74). However, the body is 'something we are, we do and we have in everyday life' and connects aspects of identity and self-management in contemporary culture (Elliott, 2009, p. 74). Within social work, attempts to reintegrate consideration of the body in practice have been most clearly developed in the work of Cameron and McDermott (2007). These authors suggest that social workers who have not been exposed to thinking about the body may enter practice with little understanding of, for example, the impact of a stroke on an older adult, who may already be a carer. An understanding of the emotional impact of intimate handling in medical settings is difficult if you have never been 'a patient'. As a young social worker, practising with older adults, I was 'taught' by listening to service users, their families and carers and in those rare moments where colleagues in the multidisciplinary team shared knowledge and wisdom beyond the biomedical facts. I am not arguing here for social work students to be taught about diseases. Rather, exposure to a sociological approach can enrich our understanding of the impact of a disabling chronic illness as incorporating elements of biographical disruption, adjustment to treatment and the longer term management of identity, relationships, human agency and self-efficacy (Charmaz, 1983) as well as the more traditional explanations in theories of grief and loss. Twigg's work in social policy is also very relevant when considering the body in the fields of health and social services. The body 'in treatment' becomes an object of attention and acted upon and is both central and marginal in social work in health care. Touch crosses border between the public sphere and the private domestic sphere with an impact on service user and carer alike (Twigg, 2006). These topics sit well alongside discussions of grief and loss.

A deeper reading of qualitative research on the experience of disability and illness can provide important reminders of human diversity and how age, gender, cultural, spirituality, social connectedness, psychological resilience and above all some degree of personal agency contribute to each person's sense of agency. These elements along with the resources and physical environment all contribute to each person's unique measure of well-being (Fouché and Martindale, 2011). The lesson is that each of us will make meaning of our experience of health and well-being in our own way.

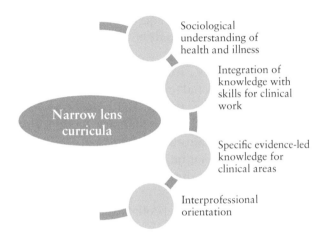

Figure 2   The narrow lens curricula

An adequate preparation for specialist practice in health care has one further specific strand I want to mention here. Practitioners in any part of the health system need to develop a dynamic understanding of the nature of interprofessional work in health care including the dynamics and issues of power and professional culture that are inherent in this context.

Social work students will be aware that interprofessional and interagency problems can cause problems in health and social services. Rivalry, status differentials and stereotypical assumptions can all impact on how people work together. It is generally argued that the conflict between disciplines is explained by the history of the development of different professions. Hall (2005) for example, describing the evolution of the health professions suggests:

> Each profession has struggled to define its identity, values, sphere of practice and role in patient care. This has led to each health care profession working within its

own silo to ensure its members ... have common experiences, values, approaches to problem-solving and language for professional tools. (Hall, 2005, p. 190)

During their professional education students not only learn the essential knowledge and skills for the practice of their profession but they also become acculturated into its values and norms. Hall and Weaver suggest that each profession might 'attract a predominance of individuals with a particular set of cognitive learning skills and styles' (Hall and Weaver, 2001, p. 873) thus influencing the problem-solving styles of different disciplines.

In recent decades health and social services have moved towards reducing the problems associated with inflexible professional territories. These changes have been intensified by the complexity of contemporary systems, the influence of service user rights, input and advocacy, which, 'whether driven by consumerist ideas or principles of social justice, required the development of responses which crossed arbitrary organisational boundaries' (Smith and Anderson, 2008, p. 760).

Interprofessional work involves three important facets: an understanding of both service user and professional experiences and contexts; clarity about different professional perspectives, theory and policies and a commitment to foster creative and collaborative interdisciplinary work focused on effective solutions to problems identified (Smith and Anderson, 2008, p. 769). Trust and respect develops with an appreciation of the roles of the other professions in health. Educators can seek opportunities to raise awareness of interprofessional work through developing case studies of particular health challenges and bringing in other professionals to model collaborative practice. This can include exploring shared decision-making among team members; the development of shared goals focussing on client/patient-centred care and knowledge of the community or client/patient group. The advancement of working across boundaries between professions, agencies and organisations is important to social workers in all fields, but it is in health where this is likely to be an everyday feature.

Conclusions

Social work education needs to provide a potent challenge to the medical paradigm and to ensure that students and beginning practitioners are well prepared to resist capture by the medical model and especially by the glamour of specialized hospital work. Exposure to wide lens content throughout the social work degree encourages the conceptualisation of the role of social workers in health care systems as an 'insider' role, enabled to advocate for social reform and policy and practice innovation. Data gained during practice on the well-being and health of citizens and communities can be used to promote social justice and effective policy change. When aiming to teach about health and well-being throughout the curriculum the educator's role is to constantly move focus between the wide lens socioeconomic and population-based views of health and the narrow lens examination of how individuals construct meaning of their own experiences of health, well-being, illness and disability. Table 1 uses chronic illness as a theme to explore curriculum themes through narrow and wide lens. These questions may be just as pertinent to acute illness as chronic illness.

Table 1 Exploring health through narrow and wide lens questions

CHRONIC ILLNESS		
Dimension	*Narrow lens questions*	*Wide lens questions*
Experience	What is this service user's experience of health and illness? How are they making meaning of issues of loss and grief?	What is the prevalence of this illness in this ethnic group, population or geographical community?
Resources	What personal, family and community resources are present or absent that may impact on their ability to face the biographical and social disruption resulting from the illness?	Do social inequalities impinge on resources for high-quality care? How does poverty impact on housing, heating, food, education, communications?
Impacts	How can he/she be supported to rebuild quality of life after a diagnosis of a chronic condition?	What is the impact of adverse features of the physical environment—water, climate, pollution, food scarcity?
Family and culture	What cultural and spiritual strengths contribute to their well-being and are there barriers to expression on these strengths in the social environment?	Who else is vulnerable here as a consequence of unequal life chances? What are the life course implications for the individual and his/her family, carers, friends and any dependants?
Strengths and risks	Is attention being paid in the health care setting to strengths as well as risk factors?	What are the barriers to accessing health care and social supports? Does structural discrimination and/or racism impact here? What community resources can be supported or developed?
Health promotion	What changes can be supported to boost resilient coping and personal and family agency?	What changes can be promoted to prevent repeated patterns of illness?
Stigma	Are there stigmatizing features associated with this illness and what impact does stigma have on well-being and self-care?	What role can education and advocacy play to raise awareness and avoid stereotyping or stigmatizing assumptions about users of particular services?

This chapter has argued that social work education should aspire to give students the ability to ask both the narrow- and wide-lens questions to enable them to respond appropriately to service users. This differs considerably from a more traditional approach of teaching students how to respond to a few key health issues or disabilities. Not only is it not feasible to teach students about every illness, but as new diseases emerge (for example consider the case of the psychosocial and human rights issues posed by growing awareness of HIV/ AIDS , SARS and so forth), social workers need the capability to respond to these and the social impacts which emerge from these. Bringing health and well-being issues into sharper focus within social work education should not be difficult, rather this change can foster creative and dynamic opportunities to develop exciting curriculum and ultimately improved outcomes for practice.

References

Ashcroft, R. (2011) 'Health and wellbeing: Starting with a critical pedagogical model', *Social Work Education*, vol. 30, no. 6, pp. 610–622.

Auerbach, C., Mason, S. E. & Heft LaPorte, H. (2007) 'Evidence that supports the value of social work in hospitals', *Social Work in Health Care*, vol. 44, pp. 17–32.

Auerbach, C. & Mason, S. E. (2010) 'The value of the presence of social work in emergency departments', *Social Work in Health Care*, vol. 49, no. 4, pp. 314–326.

Beck, U. (1992) *Risk society: Towards a new modernity*, Sage, London.

Beddoe, L. (2010) *Building professional capital: New Zealand social workers and continuing education*. Unpublished PhD thesis. (Deakin University, Victoria, Australia).

Beddoe, L. (2011a) 'Health social work: Professional identity and knowledge', *Qualitative Social Work*. doi:10.1177/1473325011415455

Beddoe, L. (2011b) 'Investing in the future: Social workers talk about research', *British Journal of Social Work*, vol. 41, no. 3, pp. 557–575.

Besthorn, F. (2003) 'Radical Ecologisms: Insights for educating social workers in ecological activism and social justice', *Critical Social Work*, 4(1). Retrieved from http://www.uwindsor.ca/criticalsocialwork/2003-volume-4-no-1

Björkenheim, J. (2007) 'Knowledge and social work in health care: The Case of Finland', *Social Work in Health Care*, vol. 44, no. 3, pp. 261–278.

Bywaters, P. & Napier, L. (2009) 'Revising social work's international policy statement on health: Process, outcomes and implications', *International Social Work*, vol. 52, no. 4, pp. 447–457.

Bywaters, P., Cowden, S., McLeod, E., Rose, S. & Singh, G. (2009) *Integrating health inequalities in social work learning and teaching*. Higher Education Academy, Social Work and Policy Digest 6.

Cabot, R. C. (1919) *Social work: Essays on the meeting-ground of doctor and social worker*. Houghton Mifflin Company, Boston; New York:

Cameron, N. & McDermott, F. (2007) *Social work and the body*. Palgrave Macmillan, Basingstoke.

Canadian Association of Social Workers (CASW) *Enhancing Interdisciplinary Collaboration in Primary Health Care Initiatives*. Retrieved 30/01/10 from http://www.casw-acts.ca/index.html

Canadian Association of Social Workers (CASW). *Preparing for change: Social work in primary health care*, November 2003. Retrieved 30/01/10 from http://www.casw-acts.ca/index.html

Charmaz, K. (1983) 'Loss of self: a fundamental form of suffering in the chronically ill', *Sociology of Health & Illness*, vol. 5, no. 2, pp. 168–195.

Clark, A. (2011) 'It is time for social workers to claim their place in Australia's health care system', *Australian Policy Online*. Retrieved 11 December 2011 from http://apo.org.au/commentary/it-time-social-workers-claim-their-place-australia%E2%80%99s-health-care-system

Coates, J. (2003) *Ecology and social work: Toward a new paradigm*. Fernwood Publishing, Halifax.

Coren, E., Iredale, W., Bywaters, P., Rutter, D. & Robinson, J. (2010) *The contribution of social work and social care to the reduction of health inequalities: Four case studies* Research Briefing 33. Retrieved from http://www.scie.org.uk/publications/briefings/briefing33/index.asp

Coren, E., Iredale, W., Rutter, D. & Bywaters, P. (2011) 'The contribution of social work and social interventions across the life course to the reduction of health inequalities: A new agenda for social work education?' *Social Work Education*, vol. 30, no. 6, pp. 594–609.

Dominelli, L. (1996) 'Deprofessionalizing social work: Anti-oppressive practice, competencies and postmodernism', *British Journal of Social Work*, vol. 26, pp. 153–175.

Elliott, A. (2009) *Contemporary Social Theory: an Introduction*, Routledge, Abingdon, Oxford.

Fouché, C. & Martindale, K. (2011) 'Work–Life Balance: Practitioner Well-Being in the Social Work Education Curriculum', *Social Work Education*, vol. 30, no. 6, pp. 675–685.

Giles, R. (2009) 'Developing a health equality imagination: Hospital practice challenges for social work priorities', *International Social Work*, vol. 52, no. 4, pp. 525–537.

Giles, R., Gould, S., Hart, C. & Swancott, J. (2007) 'Clinical priorities: Strengthening social work practice in health', *Australian Social Work*, vol. 60, no. 2, pp. 147–165.

Green, L. C. (2006) 'Pariah profession, debased discipline? An analysis of social work's low academic status and the possibilities for change', *Social Work Education*, vol. 25, no. 3, pp. 245–264.

Hall, P. (2005) 'Interprofessional teamwork: Professional cultures as barriers', *Journal of Interprofessional Care*, vol. 19, no. 2 (supp 1), pp. 188–196.

Hall, P. & Weaver, L. (2001) 'Interdisciplinary education and teamwork: A long and winding road', *Medical Education*, vol. 35, pp. 867–875.

Healy, K. (2009) 'A case of mistaken identity: The social welfare professions and New Public Management', *Journal of Sociology*, vol. 45, no. 4, pp. 401–418.

International Federation of Social Workers (2008) International Policy on Health. Retrieved 30 November 2011 from http://www.ifsw.org/en/p38000081.html

Irish Association of Social Workers (2010) Primary Care Social Work: Definition and Role. Retrieved 11 December 2011 from http://www.iasw.ie/index.php/special-interest-groups/sig-social-workers-in-primary-care

Joubert, L. (2006) 'Academic-practice partnerships in practice research: a cultural shift for health social workers', *Social Work in Health Care*, vol. 43, no. 2/3, pp. 151–162.

Keefe, R. H. (2010) 'Health disparities: A primer for public health social workers', *Social Work in Public Health*, vol. 25, no. 3–4, pp. 237–257.

Kemp, S. P. (2011) 'Recentring environment in social work practice: Necessity, opportunity, challenge', *British Journal of Social Work*, vol. 41, no. 6, pp. 1198–1210.

Littrell, J. (2008) 'The mind–body connection: Not just a theory anymore', *Social Work in Health Care*, vol. 46, no. 4, pp. 17–37.

McKinnon, J. (2008) 'Exploring the nexus between social work and the environment', *Australian Social Work*, vol. 61, no. 3, pp. 256–268.

McLeod, E. (2002) 'Social work in primary health care settings', *British Journal of Social Work*, vol. 32, no. 1, pp. 121–122.

McLeod, E. & Bywaters, P. (2002) *Social Work, Health and Equality*, Routledge, London.

Meekosha, H. & Dowse, L. (2007) 'Integrating critical disability studies into social work education and practice: An Australian perspective', *Practice*, vol. 19 no. 3, pp. 169–183.

Nilsson, D., Ryan, M. & Miller, J. (2007) 'Applying a theory of expertise in health social work administration and practice in Australia', *Social Work in Health Care*, vol. 44, no. 4, pp. 1–16.

Olgiati, V. (2006) 'Shifting heuristics in the sociological approach to professional trustworthiness: The sociology of science', *Current Sociology*, vol. 54, no. 4, pp. 533–547.

Orme, J. & Rennie, G. (2006) 'The role of registration in ensuring ethical practice', *International Social Work*, vol. 49, no. 3, pp. 333–344.

Roach-Anleu, S. L. (1992) 'The professionalisation of social work? A case study of three organisational settings', *Sociology*, vol. 26, no. 1, pp. 23–43.

Rose, S. M. & Hatzenbuehler, S. (2009) 'Embodying social class: The link between poverty, income inequality and health', *International Social Work*, vol. 52, no. 4, pp. 459–471.

Ruth, B. J., Sisco, S., Wyatt, J., Bethke, C., Bachman, S. & Markham Piper, T. (2008) 'Public health and social work: Training dual professionals for the contemporary workplace', *Public Health Reports*, vol. 123 (Supp 2), pp. 71–77.

Smith, R. & Anderson, L. (2008) 'Interprofessional learning: Aspiration or achievement?' *Social Work Education*, vol. 27, no. 7, pp. 759–776.

Social Work and Health Inequalities Network Website retrieved 11 December 2011 at http://www2.warwick.ac.uk/fac/cross_fac/healthatwarwick/research/devgroups/socialwork/swhin

Todd, A. J. (1919) *The Scientific Spirit and Social Work*, Macmillan, New York.

Turner, B. S. (1992) *Regulating Bodies: Essays in Medical Sociology*, Routledge, London; New York.

Twigg, J. (2006) *The Body in Health and Social Care*, Palgrave, Basingstoke; New York.

Union of the Physically Impaired Against Segregation and the Disability Alliance (1976) *Summary of the discussion held on 22nd November, 1975 and containing commentaries from each organisation*. London: Union of the Physically Impaired Against Segregation.

Vojak, C. (2009) 'Choosing language: Social service framing and social justice', *British Journal of Social Work*, vol. 39, no. 5, pp. 936–949.

Vourlekis, B. S., Ell, K. & Padgett, D. (2001) 'Educating social workers for health care's brave new world', *Journal of Social Work Education*, vol. 37, no. 1, pp. 177–191.

Webb, S. A. (2006) *Social work in a risk society: Social and political perspectives*, Palgrave Macmillan, New York.

Whitehead, M. (2007) 'A typology of actions to tackle social inequalities in health', *Journal of Epidemiology & Community Health*, vol. 61, no. 6, pp. 473–478.

Whiteside, M. (2004) 'The challenge of interdisciplinary collaboration in addressing the social determinants', *Australian Social Work*, vol. 57, no. 4, pp. 381–393.

World Health Organization (1986) The Ottawa Charter for Health Promotion, accessed 1 May 2011 from http://www.who.int/healthpromotion/conferences/previous/ottawa/en/.

Zapf, M. K. (2008) 'Transforming social work's understanding of person and environment: Spirituality and the "Common Ground"' *Journal of Religion & Spirituality in Social Work: Social Thought*, vol. 27, no. 1, pp. 171–181.

The Contribution of Social Work and Social Interventions Across the Life Course to the Reduction of Health Inequalities: A New Agenda for Social Work Education?

Esther Coren, Wendy Iredale, Deborah Rutter & Paul Bywaters

Inequalities in health and well-being are wide and widening and reflect the disadvantaged circumstances in which many people live. Users of personal social services in many cases already experience disadvantaged health and well-being. Social work has established experience of working with marginalised groups, and may play a role in promoting individual and community health and well-being. The value base for social work includes a focus on social justice, which may directly impact on the social determinants of health. Using four examples of social interventions across the life span, this paper considers the role that social work can play in improving the health and well-being of disadvantaged people across the life course, and the implications of this for evidence based social work practice and education.

Since the 1990s, a preoccupation with risk and its management has become central to social interventions (Bornat and Bytheway, 2010), detracting from a more holistic approach to social work practice and education (France *et al.*, 2010). Macdonald and Macdonald (2010) suggest that social work concentrates too heavily on low-probability, high-cost outcomes. Thus, social care efforts would be better placed in identifying those whose welfare is seriously compromised and seeking to address the underlying causes, rather than minimising unquantifiable risks (Gordon and Gibbons, 1998). The key challenge for social workers is to address underlying threats to well-being that may develop into risk. Thus, social work education optimally needs more focus on the range of interacting factors which contribute to an individual's health, well-being and resources, where there may be no obvious risk of immediate harm but where well-being and quality of life is threatened.

One way in which social work and social interventions might impact on the underlying causes that lead to risk is to address factors which underlie inequalities in health and well-being: the social determinants of health [Commission on the Social Determinants of Health (CSDH), 2008]. Despite continuing overall improvements in life expectancy, inequalities in UK health outcomes, for example, are wide and widening (Boyle et al., 2009), reflecting international patterns. Differences in average life expectancy between the most and least disadvantaged UK local areas increased from 9 to 11 years for men over the decade to 2001 (CSDH, 2008). Crucially, however, inequalities do not impact only on the most disadvantaged, but are reflected in a gradient across the population: 'Put simply, the higher one's social position, the better one's health is likely to be' (Marmot, 2010, p. 4), and this association is a global phenomenon (CSDH, 2008). Social services are mainly delivered to people with social and health disadvantages, a large proportion of whom are already ill and/or disabled. Social work has established experience of working with marginalised groups, and may play an important role in promoting individual and community health and well-being. Social work values include a focus on social justice, human rights and empowerment which may directly impact on the social determinants of health (Bywaters, 2009). By interrogating the role that social work can play in the health and well-being of disadvantaged people across the life course, important evidence-based recommendations for social work education can be developed.

The social determinants of health—'the circumstances in which people grow, live, work, and age, (and how they are) shaped by political, social, and economic forces'—impact on health status throughout the life span (Marmot, 2010, Preface). These determinants reflect the conditions of social life which contribute to social inequality and well-being: access to material resources and services, locality factors, education, training and employment, and individual factors such as access to social capital and the confidence or esteem to benefit from opportunities. Many users of personal social services have a lifetime history of such disadvantaged circumstances (McLeod and Bywaters, 2000; CSDH, 2008) and this may be central to their involvement with personal social services.

Implicit within this complex understanding of health, and disadvantages in health and well-being, is the acknowledgement that health cannot be reduced to physical pathology. According to the WHO (1948), health is not only the absence of disease, but a state of complete physical, mental and social well-being. Our focus is therefore the social determinants and physical, mental and social outcomes of a healthy life, and how these might be influenced by social interventions.

Poor health and well-being should be seen in terms of cumulative disadvantages across the life course (Bywaters, 2007) and the effects of early disadvantage on health and well-being may only be apparent in later life. For example, children and young people who have experienced abuse or neglect, who are disabled, or in local authority care, and their parents, are among those most likely to die prematurely as a result of poor health and unhealthy lifestyles (Davey-Smith, 2003). The health disadvantage of people with mental illnesses, who have learning disabilities or are disabled, or who are addicted to drugs or alcohol, is exacerbated because these circumstances create barriers to economic, environmental and social success, and because their physical health needs may be neglected (Michael and Richardson, 2008). As the Marmot Review (2010) argues, investment during the early years of life may be the most important priority for reducing health inequalities within a generation.

This paper discusses evidence that social work can contribute to reducing health disadvantage across the life course. Based on a preliminary synthesis of selected published research—a SCIE research briefing (Coren et al., 2010)—we demonstrate how social work and social care can impact on factors that contribute to health disadvantage and how these findings might inform social work education. We use the framework provided by the UK General Social Care Council's Codes of Practice for Social Care Workers (2010) to highlight the correspondence between social work practice and values and the promotion of health and well-being.

Review of Literature

The literature below illustrates the impact of social care and social work-led interventions on health. No studies were found which attempted to show that inequalities in health across the population as a whole were reduced. Therefore the studies reported were included because they evidenced attempts to improve the health of service users, through impact upon the social determinants of health.

Four examples of social interventions across the life span were identified: early years programmes, kinship care for children in out-of-home care, parenting programmes for parents with learning disabilities and extra care housing for older people. The literature included was international research on interventions in the developed world published in English. For further details on search methods please see SCIE (2009).

Findings

The UK General Social Care Council Codes of Practice (2010) for social care workers and employers in the UK describe expected standards of conduct and practice. We use these in the absence of a more international code of practice. However, the International Federation of Social Workers (2010) has as its priorities 'social justice, human rights and social development through the development of social work, best practices and international cooperation between social workers and their professional organisations', consistent with the UK codes.

The codes state that social workers must:

- protect the rights and promote the interests of service users and carers;
- strive to establish and maintain the trust and confidence of service users and carers;
- promote the independence of service users while protecting them as far as possible from danger or harm;
- respect the rights of service users whilst seeking to ensure that their behaviour does not harm themselves or other people;
- uphold public trust and confidence in social care services; and
- be accountable for the quality of their work and take responsibility for maintaining and improving their knowledge and skills.

We use these six key obligations as a framework for reporting evidence of the actual or potential impact of social work and social care on health disadvantage. Evidence is presented according to the four intervention types discussed above, with a table presented for each code, separated into findings and recommendations for practice development as supported in the literature.

Protect the Rights and Promote the Interests of Service Users and Carers

The research discussed in Table 1 suggests that by protecting the rights and promoting the interests of service users and carers, social care workers may impact on the social determinants of health across the life course.

Strive to Establish and Maintain the Trust and Confidence of Service Users and Carers

If service users are to benefit from services, they must have trust and confidence in services and staff. This may be particularly important for service users from minority or marginalised groups (see Table 2).

Promote the Independence of Service Users while Protecting Them as Far as Possible from Danger or Harm

The research discussed in Table 3 suggests that social care-led interventions can impact on determinants of health by promoting independence, skills, competencies and resilience across the life course.

Respect the Rights of Service Users whilst Seeking to Ensure that Their Behaviour Does Not Harm Themselves or Other People

The research discussed in Table 4 suggests that social work values, including the promotion of social justice and individual rights, are consistent with reducing the risk of harm to self and others arising from disadvantaged life circumstances.

Table 1 Protect the Rights and Promote the Interests of Service Users and Carers

Early years (EY)	Kinship care	Parents with learning disabilities (LD)	Older adults
Findings: Early years (EY) investment 'vital' to reduce health inequalities (Marmot Review, 2010).	*Findings*: For young people in out of home care, kinship care may promote better emotional/mental health outcomes compared to other forms of care (Farmer, 2009; Winokur *et al.*, 2009).	*Findings*: Women with LD have less access to maternity care choices (Campion, 1996).	*Findings*: Social care may impact on health outcomes by improving living conditions. Extra care housing (ECH) may offer better quality of life than elsewhere (Croucher *et al.*, 2006; Brooker and Wooley, 2006).
EY programmes improve maternal and child health. Sure Start improved outcomes (breast feeding, baby massage, improved child confidence) (Northrop *et al.*, 2008).	Stein (2009) suggests that placement stability for children aged 11 + is central to well-being, school satisfaction and general happiness: kinship care associated with greater placement stability.	Parents with LD may experience difficulties accessing resources (Tagg and Kenny, 2006).	ECH found to reduce residents' hospital stays and severity of diagnosed mental illnesses (Croucher, 2007; Brooker *et al.*, 2009).
Sure Start home visits improved family health and parental confidence (NESS, 2001, 2006). Parents with LD may not reach local service thresholds, and only come to services' attention if children perceived as in need/at risk (Ward and Tarleton, 2007).			Tenants who engaged with community activities in ECH found life more stimulating (Evans and Vallelly, 2007; Evans, 2008).
Sure Start children had improved learning skills/attitudes; better social development (Ofsted, 2009).			Less known about meeting needs of specific groups, e.g. those with sensory impairments/dementia (Bernard *et al.*, 2007; Dutton, 2009).
Adults who received pre-school programme achieved higher academic scores (Campbell *et al.*, 2002; Hill *et al.*, 2003; Melhuish and Office, 2004; Blok *et al.*, 2005).			
Sure Start increased confidence, parenting skills, child–parent bonds, social capital and empowerment (NESS Research Team, 2001, 2006, 2008; Bagley and Ackerley, 2006; Anning *et al.*, 2007; Allen, 2008).			

Table 2 Strive to Establish and Maintain Trust and Confidence of Service Users and Carers

Early years	Kinship care	Parents with learning disabilities	Older adults
Findings: Parents of disabled children may find accessing Sure Start difficult (Pinney, 2007). Mainly mothers as men may feel uncomfortable (Pearson and Thurston, 2006).	*Findings*: Kinship carers often paid far less than non-kinship foster carers and offered minimal support; level/-type of support for kinship care placements varies geographically (Aldgate and McIntosh, 2006).	*Findings*: Despite policy, parents with LD feel judged by professionals not supported (Olsen and Wates, 2003; Tagg and Kenny, 2006) and fear removal of children. Parents often socially excluded and may depend on statutory agencies for support (McGraw *et al.*, 2002). To avoid labelling as 'in need', parents may reject not seek help (Ward and Tarleton, 2007).	*Findings*: Support varies between providers. Differences in scheme success may depend on rural/urban location (Easterbrook and Vallelly, 2008).
Recommendations: Creating staff teams from varied social groups and striving to reach all eligible families requires improved inter-agency working (NESS, 2005). Involving minority staff in designing services may promote minority groups' access (Craig, 2007).	*Recommendations*: Greater equity in support required to improve kin confidence to take on foster care and avoid financial hardship.	*Recommendations*: To promote confidence, service focus should actively shift from judgement to support.	*Recommendations*: Older people's care should not be geographically dependent; access to social/leisure facilities may be especially important in rural areas (Allardice, 2005).

Table 3 Promote Independence of Service Users while Protecting Them as Far as Possible from Danger or Harm

Early years	Kinship care	Parents with learning disabilities	Older adults
Findings: Evaluation literature supports community development as 'added value'. Supportive partnerships, social and local community networks can be protective and help parents with child-rearing (Cowley, 1999). Evidence of increased 'community spirit' with Sure Start parents working together to improve local communities (NESS, 2001). Local variation in degree to which parents' mutual support and volunteering generated community empowerment (NESS, 2001). *Recommendations*: Research should assess the role of process factors, e.g. style or management of service delivery, in achieving such outcomes, to enable service development to optimize potential.	*Findings*: Kinship carers appear financially disadvantaged (Aldgate and McIntosh, 2006). Under-resourcing may exacerbate health inequalities: without adequate support, kinship carers (often grandparents) and young people have increased risk of disadvantaged health/well-being outcomes. (Aldgate and McIntosh, 2006).	*Findings*: Parents with LD may develop independence through skills training (Sheerin, 1998; Tagg and Kenny, 2006). Indications that parenting skills can improve through self-instructional pictorial child-care cards (Feldman *et al.*, 1997; Feldman and Case, 1999); nutrition and feeding training (Feldman *et al.*, 1997); group learning (Heinz and Grant, 2003), and home-based training (Llewellyn and McConnell, 2002; Mildon *et al.*, 2008; Wade *et al.*, 2008). Parents with LD may have few supportive friends/neighbours relationships (Llewellyn, 2002).	*Findings*: Extra care housing may increase feelings of safety and protection whilst maintaining independence, offering social, recreational and medical provisions 'in-house', improving safety and sense of community. Thus, retirement villages can improve both independence and security (Bernard *et al.*, 2007; Croucher, 2007; Brooker *et al.*, 2009).

30

Table 4 Respect the Rights of Service Users whilst Seeking to Ensure that Their Behaviour Does Not Harm Themselves or Other People

Early years	Kinship care	Parents with learning disabilities	Older adults
Findings: EY care may not reach groups most at risk: most vulnerable may be hardest to reach (Barlow *et al.*, 2005).	*Findings*: Kinship carers disadvantaged compared to others, including limitations to freedom for children/-carers; issues for older carers coping with behaviour of young people; lack of agency support; overcrowding; carer ill health; less thorough assessments than for non-familial carers; less strict monitoring, lower reunification (Aldgate and McIntosh, 2006).	*Findings*: Parents may lack skills/-knowledge re: sex education, child health, safety and development (Campion, 1996; James, 2004) so may engage in behaviour which could impact on parent/child. Parents can improve child care and safety through audiovisual self-instructional handbooks (Feldman *et al.*, 1997; Feldman and Case, 1999) or home-based interventions (Llewellyn *et al.*, 2003). Parenting programmes may only be offered in extreme cases where children are at risk (Sheerin, 1998).	*Findings*: ECH residents may experience lower health risks than those elsewhere, e.g. Vallelly *et al.* (2006) found that residents have most health care needs met in-house, with more opportunity to access GP home visits/preventive services, e.g. physiotherapists or chiropodists.
Recommendations: Creating a team from a diverse population, and striving to reach all eligible families requires more effective inter-agency working (NESS, 2006). 'Hard to reach' groups, e.g. minority ethnic communities, disabled people and caregivers, people with learning difficulties, young mothers and new service users more likely to engage if they receive home visits (NESS, 2006; Pearson and Thurston, 2006).	*Recommendations*: Challenge is to support kinship placements, reducing risk factors to enable opportunities that equip children for successful future (Aldgate and McIntosh, 2006).	*Recommendations*: Services should provide preventative care, supporting parents where children not identified as 'at risk' (Sheerin, 1998). Multi-agency collaboration optimal (Sheerin, 1998; Tymchuk, 1999).	*Recommendations*: ECH must balance quality of life with risk management. Overcautious approaches can limit opportunities for social interaction, particularly for residents with impaired mobility (Evans and Vallelly, 2007).

Uphold Public Trust and Confidence in Social Care Services

The research discussed in Table 5 suggests that social care work can improve outcomes for, and protect, marginalised and vulnerable groups, which is consistent with the public expectation of social welfare.

Be Accountable for the Quality of Their Work and Take Responsibility for Maintaining and Improving Their Knowledge and Skills

Social work and social care workers are expected to be accountable for improving knowledge and skills, which requires access to best possible evidence. However, there are gaps in the literature that suggest more evidence is needed to understand the potential impact of social work on health inequalities. Table 6 outlines some gaps in literature identified by this overview.

Discussion

The Marmot Review of health inequalities policy in England (Marmot, 2010, p. 159) states that adult social care, 'makes a significant contribution to health and to health inequalities', while also emphasising the importance of children's services to health. The Review asserts that access to holistic social care services is a health inequalities issue and that sustained, adequate funding, 'the greater integration of health and social care, and joint action on health inequalities' is required to underpin this. However, it cannot be assumed that well intentioned preventive action which benefits some groups within the population will necessarily reduce *inequalities* in health (Capewell and Graham, 2010) and so evidence is needed of the impact of social interventions on the distribution of health outcomes. The aims of this paper were to pilot a review of such evidence and consider the implications for social work and social care education, research, and practice. The UK General Social Care Council's *Codes of Practice for Social Care Workers* (2010) was adopted as a framework for reporting reviews covering four examples of social work and social care practice across the life course.

Four broad conclusions can be drawn from these reviews.

Firstly, there is currently little or no conclusive evidence at the population level of the impact of social work or social care interventions on health inequalities, because such research hardly exists. Although this may be partially due to methodological and resourcing difficulties, we suspect it is largely due to a lack of focus on this aspect of practice. We therefore had to draw inferences from studies of the health impact of interventions targeted at disadvantaged populations, or consider the impact of interventions on aspects of the social determinants of health. The development of an epidemiological approach within social work and social care research could be valuable.

Secondly, the reviews have demonstrated the relevance of social work and social care interventions for promoting physical and mental health, preventing illness and helping people to build and maintain independence and life skills that improve outcomes

Table 5 Uphold Public Trust and Confidence in Social Care Services

Early years	Kinship care	Parents with learning disabilities	Older adults
Findings: Families' engagement with Sure Start negatively associated with disadvantage and risk, i.e. under-representation of teen parents, lone parents and unemployed (Siraj-Blatchford and Siraj-Blatchford, 2009). Identified barriers to uptake were: transport, cost, language and inaccurate perception (e.g. thinking Sure Start was just for 'disadvantaged people'; Coe et al., 2008). *Recommendations*: Implications for promotion, funding and staffing (see earlier sections)	*Findings*: Research shows kinship care to be beneficial, but carers may be inhibited due to financial hardship and lack of agency support (Aldgate and McIntosh, 2006). *Recommendations*: Kinship carers need stronger support and funding to enable better opportunity for placement stability (Broad, 2007).	*Findings*: Despite high rates of child removal from LD parents, investment in to promote effective parenting low (Booth and Booth, 1999). Environmental factors, e.g. poverty, lack of support to understand early development needs, disadvantage parents with LD (Tagg and Kenny, 2006). *Recommendations*: Advocacy alone will not relieve pressures that undermine parents' coping (Tagg and Kenny, 2006). Presumption of incompetence by professionals, including fixed ideas about options for children; tension between policing and enabling roles; services de-skilling parents by taking over responsibilities; blaming victims rather than addressing deficiencies in system; lack of trust; and services offering conflicting advice (Booth and Booth, 1999; Ward and Tarleton, 2007).	*Findings*: Dawson et al. (2006) found that the most influential factor promoting development of ECH was good partnerships between social services, housing departments and older people. *Recommendations*: Planning, design and management of ECH, should prioritise social well-being of residents (Evans and Vallelly, 2007). Staff training/remuneration is key to developing integrated, responsive services, especially where needs are diverse (Allardice, 2005).

33

Table 6 Be Accountable for the Quality of Their Work and Take Responsibility for Maintaining and Improving Their Knowledge and Skills

Early years	Kinship care	Parents with learning disabilities	Older adults
Findings: To reduce inequality of access, more should be done to address barriers to accessing services. Variation in service use by different minority groups, genders, disabilities and regional variations need further exploration. Social workers may play a role in improving access to services by disadvantaged families.	*Findings*: Research suggests social workers could reduce inequality by advocating for equality of support between kin and non-kin foster carers. Literature on kinship care focuses on behaviour and placement stability rather than health and well-being. Evaluations needed of health/well-being outcomes for young people and kinship carers compared to standard foster care.	*Findings*: Evidence shows that interventions for parents with LD may improve parenting skills and promote parenting by parents. But, interventions cannot address structural issues: poverty, social isolation and poor service provision that may prevent parents with LD achieving equal care. Research assessed does not address regional variation. Practitioners manage dual roles: supporting parents and monitoring parenting capacity. Research needed to address inclusion in different regions or among groups that may be further marginalised due to, e.g. ethnicity, religion, physical or sensory disability.	*Findings*: Existing evidence on housing needs of older people from ethnic minorities relates mainly to sheltered accommodation (Jones, 2006), with little provision for ethnic-specific ECH. Consideration should be given to mixed environments and to balancing integration with religious groups' desire for separate provision (Allardice, 2005; Jones, 2008). Knowledge of how to meet needs of older people from minority groups remains limited, and is a gap in UK evidence base (Croucher *et al.*, 2006). Some suggest that the evidence base for ECH does not support the claim that it provides a fully supportive environment, and argue for further research (Cantley and Cook, 2006).

related to the social determinants of health. These examples reinforce the general assertions of the Marmot Review (Marmot, 2010) that social care services contribute to healthier outcomes for disadvantaged people.

Thirdly, the reviews highlight the potential damage which may arise when social work or social care interventions do not adequately address the health dimensions of people's lives, including social determinants of health, such as housing, income and life skills. Failure to reach potential beneficiaries of services (fathers, or minority ethnic parents, for example), or to provide parallel support to kinship and non-kinship carers, exacerbates the unfair distribution of health and other life chances. The limited evidence which could be found which evaluated social care interventions aimed directly at service users' health is another marker of a lack of attention being paid to this in current practice and research.

Fourthly, to alter this requires greater focus in social work and social care education on the centrality of social aspects of physical and mental health in service users' lives. Three models for integrating teaching on health inequalities in social work education have been outlined in a recent digest of the Social Work and Social Policy Subject Centre of the Higher Education Academy (SWAP) in England (Bywaters *et al.*, 2009):

- *Permeation*: spreading learning about health inequalities throughout the curriculum in college and practice settings;
- *Focused health modules*: teaching about health in a discrete module or modules, taking a health inequalities perspective; and
- *Interprofessional modules*: teaching about health inequalities as a core element in interprofessional modules.

Such a shift in research, practice and education requires a policy context which current trends in England make less likely. The social care sector is not resourced to address the core social determinants of health and well-being; in particular, incomes, housing, and aspects of access to opportunities. For example, programmes aimed at supporting parents cannot compensate for low incomes and environmental deficiencies. Unsupported kinship carers, often elderly and on low incomes, do not have the same level of material support as their paid counterparts, and the continuity, stability and attachment they can offer may therefore be compromised. Reduced budgets and increased caseloads within professional social work have discouraged involvement in debt counselling, community engagement and other social determinants of healthy living. Moreover, the current UK coalition government's economic policies herald substantial cuts in local authority finances and health care funding, as well as approaches to social policy which emphasise greater targeting [for example, in Children's Centres (HM Treasury, 2010)]. These policies are unlikely to support social workers to consider the structural risk factors in service users' lives, or to encourage population based interventions, despite evidence of potential cost savings in the longer term (Aked *et al.*, 2009). However, social work education and practice should continue to use its unique perspective to highlight the failures of policy which sustain inequalities in health outcomes, with particular effect within marginalised groups.

The sector should promote service delivery approaches that reduce inequalities and advocate for individuals and populations caught in lifelong cycles of disadvantage. Recognising health as a central dimension in service users' lives and health disadvantage as a universal focus for social work intervention is the key starting point.

Acknowledgements

This paper is based on work funded and commissioned by the Social Care Institute for Excellence (Coren *et al.*, 2010). The views expressed in this paper reflect the individual views of the authors rather than those of the SCIE. The work also received institutional support from Canterbury Christ Church University. The authors gratefully acknowledge assistance from Manuela Thomae of Canterbury Christ Church University at the final draft stage.

References

Aked, J., Steuer, N., Lawlor, E. & Sprat, S. (2009) *Backing the Future: Why Investing in Children is Good for Us All*, New Economics Foundation and Action for Children, London.

Aldgate, J. & McIntosh, M. (2006) *Looking After the Family: A Study of Children Looked After in Kinship Care in Scotland*, Social Work Inspection Agency, Edinburgh.

Allardice, J. (2005) *A 2020 Vision for Housing and Car*, Jane Allardice Communications Limited, Essex [online]. Available at: http://www.hanover.org.uk/PDF/2020_vision%20report.pdf.

Allen, B. L. (2008) 'Evaluating Sure Start, Head Start, and Early Head Start: finding their signals amidst methodological static', *Journal for the Early Intervention Field*, vol. 11, no. 2, pp. 110–132.

Anning, A., Stuart, J., Nicholls, M., Goldthorpe, J. & Morley, A. (2007) *Understanding Variations in Effectiveness amongst Sure Start Local Programmes*, Research Report NESS/2007/FR/024, Department for Education and Skills, London [online]. Available at: http://www.dcsf.gov.uk/everychildmatters/_download/?id=4754.

Bagley, C. & Ackerley, C. L. (2006) '"I am much more than just a mum": social capital, empowerment and Sure Start', *Journal of Education Policy*, vol. 21, no. 6, pp. 717–734.

Barlow, J., Kirkpatrick, S., Stewart-Brown, S. & Davis, H. (2005) 'Hard to reach or out of reach? Reasons why women refuse to take part in early interventions', *Children and Society*, vol. 19, pp. 199–210.

Bernard, M., Bartlam, B. & Sim, J. (2007) 'Housing and care for older people—life in an English purpose-built retirement village', *Ageing and Society*, vol. 27, pp. 555–578.

Blok, H., Fukkink, R. G., Gebhardt, E. C. & Leseman, P. P. M. (2005) 'The relevance of delivery mode and other programme characteristics for the effectiveness of early childhood intervention', *International Journal of Behavioural Development*, vol. 291, no. 1, pp. 35–47.

Booth, T. & Booth, W. (1999) 'Parents together: action research and advocacy support for parents with learning difficulties', *Health and Social Care in the Community*, vol. 7, no. 6, pp. 464–474.

Bornat, J. & Bytheway, B. (2010) 'Perceptions and presentations of living with everyday risk in later life', *British Journal of Social Work*, vol. 40, pp. 1118–1134.

Boyle, P. J., Norman, P. & Popham, F. (2009) 'Social mobility: evidence that it can widen health inequalities', *Social Science and Medicine*, vol. 68, pp. 1835–1842.

Broad, B. (2007) 'Kinship care: what works? Who cares?', *Social Work and Social Sciences Review*, vol. 13, no. 1, pp. 59–74.

Brooker, D. & Wooley, R. (2006) *Enriching Opportunities: Unlocking Potential: Searching for the Keys*, University of Bradford, Bradford Dementia Group, Bradford.

Brooker, D. J., Argyle, E. & Clancy, D. (2009) 'The mental health needs of people living in extra care housing', *Journal of Care Services Management*, vol. 3, no. 3, pp. 295–309.

Bywaters, P. (2007) 'Understanding the lifecourse', in *Social Work: A Companion to Learning*, eds P. Bywaters & K. Postle, Sage, London.

Bywaters, P. (2009) 'Tackling inequalities in health: a global challenge for social work', *British Journal of Social Work*, vol. 39, no. 2, pp. 353–367.

Bywaters, P., Cowden, S., McLeod, E., Rose, S. & Singh, G. (2009) 'Integrating health inequalities in social work learning and teaching', in *SWAP Digest 6*, SWAP, Southampton.

Campbell, F. A., Ramey, C. T., Pungello, E., Sparling, J. & Miller-Johnson, S. (2002) 'Early childhood education: young adult outcomes from the Abecedarian Project', *Applied Developmental Science*, vol. 6, no. 1, pp. 42–57.

Campion, M. T. (1996) 'Right from the start: maternity services for people with learning disabilities', *Disability, Pregnancy and Parenthood International*, vol. 16, pp. 6–7.

Cantley, C. & Cook, M. (2006) *A Report on the Evaluation of Moor Allerton Care Centre*, Dementia North, University of Northumbria.

Capewell, S. & Graham, H. (2010) 'Will cardiovascular disease prevention widen health inequalities?', *PLoS Med*, vol. 7, no. 8, e1000320.DOI: 10.1371/journal.pmed.1000320.

Coe, C., Gibson, A. & Spencer, M. (2008) 'Sure Start: voices of the "hard-to-reach"', *Care Health and Development*, vol. 34, no. 4, pp. 447–453.

Commission on Social Determinants of Health (CSDH) (2008) *Closing the Gap in a Generation: Health Equity through Action on the Social Determinants of Health*, Final Report of the Commission on Social Determinants of Health, World Health Organisation, Geneva.

Coren, E., Iredale, W., Bywaters, P., Rutter, D. & Robinson (2010) *SCIE Research Briefing 33: The Contribution of Social Work and Social Care to the Reduction of Health Inequalities: Four Case Studies* [online]. Available at: http://www.scie.org.uk/publications/briefings/briefing33/index.asp.

Cowley, S. (1999) 'Early interventions: evidence for implementing Sure Start', *Community Practitioner*, vol. 72, no. 6, pp. 162–165.

Craig, G. (2007) *Sure Start and Black and Minority Ethnic Populations*, Department for Education and Skills, Nottingham.

Croucher, K. (2007) *Comparative Evaluations of Models of Housing with Care for Later Life*, Joseph Rowntree Foundation, London.

Croucher, K., Hicks, L. & Jackson, K. (2006) *Housing with Care for Later Life: A Literature Review*, Joseph Rowntree Foundation, London.

Davey-Smith, G. (2003) *Health Inequalities: Lifecourse Approaches*, The Policy Press, Bristol.

Dawson, L., Williams, J. & Netten, A. (2006) 'Extra care housing: is it really an option for older people?', *Housing Care and Support*, vol. 9, no. 2, pp. 23–29.

Dutton, R. (2009) *Extra Care Housing and People with Dementia: What Do We Know About What Works Regarding the Built and Social Environment, and the Provision of Care and Support? A Scoping Review of the Literature 1998–2008*, Housing and Dementia Research Consortium, London.

Easterbrook, L. & Vallelly, S. (2008) *Is it That Time Already? Extra Care Housing at the End of Life: A Policy-into-Practice Evaluation*, Housing 21.

Evans, S. (2008) *Social Well-being in Extra Care Housing*, Care Services Improvement Partnership, Housing Learning and Improvement Network.

Evans, S. & Vallelly, S. (2007) *Best Practice in Promoting Social Well-being in Extra Care Housing— A Literature Review*, Joseph Rowntree Foundation, York.

Farmer, E. (2009) 'How do placements in kinship care compare with those in non-kin foster care: placement patterns, progress and outcomes', *Child and Family Social Work*, vol. 14, no. 3, pp. 331–342.

Feldman, M. A. & Case, L. (1999) 'Teaching child-care and safety skills to parents with intellectual disabilities through self-learning', *Journal of Intellectual and Developmental Disability*, vol. 24, no. 1, pp. 27–44.

Feldman, M. A., Garrick, M. & Case, L. (1997) 'The effects of parent training on weight gain of nonorganic-failure-to-thrive children of parents with intellectual disabilities', *Journal on Developmental Disabilities*, vol. 5, no. 1, pp. 47–61.

France, A., Freiberg, K. & Homel, R. (2010) 'Beyond risk factors: towards a holistic prevention paradigm for children and young people', *British Journal of Social Work*, vol. 40, pp. 1192–1210.

General Social Care Council (GSCC) (2010) *Codes of Practice for Social Care Workers*, GSCC, London.

Gordon, D. & Gibbons, J. (1998) 'Placing children on child protection registers: risk indicators and Local Authority differences', *British Journal of Social Work*, vol. 28, pp. 423–436.

Heinz, L. C. & Grant, P. R. (2003) 'A process evaluation of a parenting group for parents with intellectual disabilities', *Evaluation and Program Planning*, vol. 26, no. 3, pp. 263–274.

Hill, J., Brooks-Gunn, J. & Waldfogel, J. (2003) 'Sustained effects of high participation in an early intervention for low birth weight premature infants', *Developmental Psychology*, vol. 39, no. 4, pp. 730–744.

HM Treasury (2010) *Spending Review 2010*, The Stationery Office, London.

International Federation for Social Workers (IFSW) (2010) *Welcome to ISFW | Human Rights Day 2010 | Speak Up Stop Discrimination* [online]. Available at: www.ifsw.org.

James, H. (2004) 'Promoting effective working with parents with learning disabilities', *Child Abuse Review*, vol. 13, no. 1, pp. 31–41.

Jones, A. (2006) *Beyond Sheltered Accommodation—A Review of Extra Care Housing and Care Home Provision for BME Elders*, Department of Health, London.

Jones, A. (2008) *Meeting the Sheltered and Extra Care Housing Needs of Black and Minority Ethnic Older People*, Race Equality Foundation, London.

Llewellyn, G. (2002) 'Home-based programmes for parents with intellectual disabilities: lessons from practice', *Journal of Applied Research in Intellectual Disabilities*, vol. 15, no. 4, pp. 341–353.

Llewellyn, G. & McConnell, D. (2002) 'Mothers with learning difficulties and their support networks', *Journal of Intellectual Disability Research*, vol. 46, no. 1, pp. 17–34.

Llewellyn, G., McConnell, D., Honey, A., Mayes, R. & Russo, D. (2003) 'Promoting health and home safety for children of parents with intellectual disability: a randomized controlled trial', *Research in Developmental Disabilities*, vol. 24, no. 6, pp. 405–431.

Macdonald, G. & Macdonald, K. (2010) 'Safeguarding: a case for intelligent risk management', *British Journal of Social Work*, vol. 40, no. 4, pp. 1174–1191.

Marmot, M. (2010) *Fair Society, Healthy Lives: Strategic Review of Health Inequalities in England Post 2010*, Department of Health, London.

McGraw, S., Ball, K. & Clark, A. (2002) 'The effect of group intervention on the relationships of parents with intellectual disabilities', *Journal of Applied Research in Intellectual Disabilities*, vol. 15, no. 4, pp. 354–366.

McLeod, E. & Bywaters, P. (2000) *Social Work, Equality and Health*, Routledge, London.

Melhuish, E. C. & Office, L. N. A. (2004) *A Literature Review of the Impact of Early Years Provision upon Young Children, with Emphasis Given to Children from Disadvantaged Backgrounds: Report to the Comptroller and Auditor General*, National Audit Office, London.

Michael, J. & Richardson, A. (2008) 'Healthcare for all: the independent inquiry into access to healthcare for people with learning disabilities', *Tizard Learning Disability Review*, vol. 13, no. 4, pp. 28–34.

Mildon, R., Wade, C. & Matthews, J. (2008) 'Considering the contextual fit of an intervention for families headed by parents with an intellectual disability: an exploratory study', *Journal of Applied Research in Intellectual Disabilities*, vol. 21, no. 4, pp. 377–387.

NESS Research Team (2001) *The Impact of Sure Start—One Year On*, DCSF, London.

NESS Research Team (2005) *Implementing Sure Start Local Programmes: An In-depth Study*, DCSF, London.

NESS Research Team (2006) *Empowering Parents in Sure Start Local Programmes*, DCSF, London.

NESS Research Team (2008) *The Impact of Sure Start Local Programmes on Three-Year-Olds and Their Families*, DCSF, London.

Northrop, M., Pittam, G. & Caan, W. (2008) 'The expectations of families and patterns of participation in a Trailblazer Sure Start', *Community Practitioner*, vol. 81, no. 2, pp. 24–28.

Ofsted (2009) *The Impact of Integrated Services on Children and Their Families in Sure Start Children's Centres*, Ofsted, London.

Olsen, R. & Wates, M. (2003) *Disabled Parents: Examining Research Assumptions*, Research in Practice, Totnes.

Pearson, C. & Thurston, M. (2006) 'Understanding mothers' engagement with antenatal parent education services: a critical analysis of a local Sure Start service', *Children and Society*, vol. 20, no. 5, pp. 348–359.

Pinney, A. (2007) *A Better Start: Children and Families with Special Needs and Disabilities in Sure Start Local Programmes*, DCSF, London.

Sheerin, F. (1998) 'Parents with learning disabilities: a review of the literature', *Journal of Advanced Nursing*, vol. 28, no. 1, pp. 126–133.

Siraj-Blatchford, I. & Siraj-Blatchford, J. (2009) *Improving Children's Attainment Through a Better Quality of Family-based Support for Early Learning*, Knowledge Review, Centre for Excellence and Outcomes in Children and Young People's Services, England.

Social Care Institute for Excellence (SCIE) (2009) *SCIE Research Briefings: Guidance*, Social Care Institute for Excellence, London [online]. Available at: http://www.scie.org.uk/publications/briefings/files/researchbriefingguidance2009.pdf.

Stein, M. (2009) *Quality Matters in Children's Services—Messages from Research*, Jessica Kingsley, London.

Tagg, L. & Kenny, G. (2006) 'Family nursing and parents who have a learning disability', *Paediatric Nursing*, vol. 18, no. 2, pp. 14–18.

Tymchuk, A. J. (1999) 'Moving towards integration of services for parents with intellectual disabilities', *Journal of Intellectual and Developmental Disability*, vol. 24, no. 1, pp. 59–74.

Vallelly, S., Evans, S., Frear, T. & Means, R. (2006) *Opening Doors to Independence: A Longitudinal Study Exploring the Contribution of Extra Care Housing to the Care and Support of People with Dementia*, Housing 21, Housing Corporation, London.

Wade, C., Llewellyn, G. & Matthews, J. (2008) 'Review of parent training interventions for parent with intellectual disability', *Journal of Applied Research in Intellectual Disabilities*, vol. 21, no. 4, pp. 351–366.

Ward, L. & Tarleton, B. (2007) 'Sinking or swimming? Supporting parents with learning disabilities and their children', *Learning Disability Review*, vol. 12, no. 2, pp. 22–32.

Winokur, M., Holtan, A. & Valentine, D. (2009) 'Kinship care for the safety, permanency, and well-being of children removed from the home for maltreatment', *Cochrane Database of Systematic Reviews*, no. 1, Art no. CD006546, DOI: 10.1002/14651858.CD006546.pub2.

World Health Organisation (WHO) (1948) *Constitution*, World Health Organisation, Geneva.

Health and Wellbeing: Starting with a Critical Pedagogical Model

Rachelle Ashcroft

There are many views on what constitutes health and wellbeing. What emerge are varying—and at times competing—discourses and recommended approaches for practice. Knowledge of these varying perspectives and the skills to critically assess their compatibility with social work values provides tools to social workers to assist in determining how to shape practice in a way that best focuses on health and wellbeing. A pedagogical model is reviewed that includes an overview of the six most dominant health paradigms: biomedicine, public health, biopsychosocial, social determinants of health, political economy, and holism.

Introduction

As a social worker in various Canadian health settings, I have often reflected on how to best approach health and wellbeing within my practice. As an academic, I have spent much time thinking about the larger forces shaping my practice as well as the many ways that health and wellbeing are approached. As an educator, I have considered how to best prepare students to meet this challenge in complex practice settings. There are many views on what constitutes health and wellbeing, thus what emerges are varying—and at times competing—discourses and recommended approaches for practice. Knowledge of these varying perspectives and the skills to critically assess their compatibility with social work values provides tools and develops critical thinking skills in preparation for a practice that attends to health issues, directly and indirectly. This article explores the benefits of adopting a critical pedagogical model for social work education in health that includes a brief identification of the most influential paradigms that shape approaches to health.

The World Health Organization (WHO) defines health as 'a state of complete physical, mental and social well being and not merely the absence of disease or infirmity' (World Health Organization, 1992). My own view of health is compatible with the WHO; that threats to physiological health are increasingly derived from multifaceted interactions among political, sociological, environmental, psychological, and biological factors. Acknowledging that health extends beyond the physiological is not new for social work. However, the meaning of health can differ from one social group to the next, between individuals (Brown, 1998; Commers, 2002), and in the various contexts that social workers find themselves practicing. Differences in how health is understood and approached in practice are influenced by the overarching paradigm guiding not just social work, but all who fall within that social group. The inclusion of a curriculum that critically explores influential health paradigms, related social groups, and the emerging approaches to health is not to negate social work's unique lens of the person-in-environment. Like Dewees and Lax (2008), this approach is to 'promote a *social work* response that sustains the profession's grounding' (p. 95) by critically examining how to best promote health and wellbeing with consideration of the influences that shape the overall approaches to health. The intent of this pedagogical approach is to best prepare social work to recognize how and why these differences in how health is understood emerge, thus arming social work with skills and tools to best determine the appropriate means of intervention.

Paradigms

Gaining a better understanding of social work in health requires the identification and deconstruction of the larger forces that shape practice. My use of the term *paradigm* is informed by Kuhn (1996) who uses it in a way that 'stands for the entire constellation of beliefs, values, techniques, and so on shared by the members of a given community' (p. 175). The health community is broad and complex with social workers in health often within a community comprised of diverse backgrounds and perspectives. Theory-making and research methodologies that guide practice are developed upon paradigms (Payne, 2005). Thus, there are various forces in health that impact on social work discourses—a term that refers to the 'political assumptions, linguistics, and attitudes' (Larson, 2008, p. 45) incorporated by way of paradigmatic influences.

What is recommended is that social work adopts a pedagogical model that provides knowledge and skills to critically understand and assess the differences and variations in health paradigms. In a way, this model is inspired by a systems approach because it provides social work with a broader understanding of their environment and the complex system of health. According to Meadows (1999), 'paradigms are the sources of systems. From shared social agreements about the nature of reality, come system goals and information flows … and everything else about systems' (p. 18).

Critical Pedagogy

What this model proposes is to critically engage social work students in the differences that emerge in health discourse. Critical thought and engagement with the differing beliefs and approaches has a potential to increase our understanding and strengthen our actions (Skelton, 2005; McArthur, 2010) in all the health related contexts in which social workers are employed. Critical pedagogy involves an action oriented agenda 'through education and throughout society' (McArthur, 2010, p. 493). The intent of this pedagogical model is to challenge students to critically consider the variations and differences in how health is understood and approached. The goal is that, once in practice, social workers will use the knowledge and acquired skills in action to have the greatest impact on individual and collective health and wellbeing. Adopting a critical pedagogical model embraces the 'belief that education and society are intrinsically inter-related and that the fundamental purpose of education is the improvement of social justice for all' (McArthur, 2010, p. 493).

One objective in social work education is to convey knowledge that helps students engage in critical reflection about power and inequality, or what Freire refers to as conscientization (Freire, 1973; Millstein, 1997; Lavoie, 2001). 'The conscientientiza-tion ... that occurs is important in creating an impetus for change and for building confidence in one's own power to bring about that change' (Lavoie, 2001, p. 31). The use of a deconstruction process as a pedagogical tool fosters critical thinking about larger social and political processes while enabling a sense of critical thought about one's own situation as a social worker. The knowledge and skills gained in this manner will enable social workers to be able to determine the best approaches towards health with individuals, communities, and larger populations.

Furthermore, this approach interconnects micro, meso, and macro level structures thus offering a rich understanding of the pathways to health and wellness. This is an important inclusion in a critical pedagogical health model as these various levels all impact on one another: 'A movement such as critical pedagogy that wishes to effect change must consider them all' (McArthur, 2010, p. 494).

Providing social work students with an understanding of influential values, historical and social processes that shape health paradigms, provides them with the critical lens necessary to help determine the most effective intervention strategies to employ in their practice. In my own education of theories and social institutions, Dr Martha Kuwee Kumsa—a significant academic mentor of mine—would frequently remind us that institutions 'didn't just fall from the sky'. The message within Dr Kumsa's teachings is an inherent component within this pedagogical model; although some health institutions and practices may be deeply rooted, change is possible.

Paradigm analysis encourages examination of the basic beliefs and assumptions that define and organize the nature of the world (Nelson *et al.*, 2001; Guba and Lincoln, 2005). Developing curriculum based on a paradigm deconstruction model is inclusive of influential historical factors, underlying values and epistemology, assumptions of health, policy, and intervention strategies. Waldram's (2004) assertion 'that there is a political dimension to healing today is without question' (p. 299), further emphasizes the need to delve deeper into existing paradigms in order to unravel the values and beliefs that shape and guide social work discourse in health and wellbeing. Influential health paradigms are broad umbrellas that guide and are shaped by a menagerie of people. Highlighting how social work has evolved and is shaped by the larger health paradigms can be done with the use of a social work-specific typology.

Typology of Social Work

One example of a social work-specific typology that can be included in this critical paradigm model is Payne's (2005, 2006) typology of social work. Payne (2005, 2006) illustrates three primary views of social work; each of these views outlines a particular way in which this interaction takes form: 'Every bit of practice, all practice ideas, all social work agency organization and all welfare policy is a rubbing up of three views of social work against each other' (Payne, 2006, p. 12). This is not to imply that all of social work practice is homogenous and equally contains these various views. The representation of the three views can emerge differently in practice, with emphasis being on one view more so than another.

The three views of social work include: the therapeutic view (reflexive-therapeutic), the social order view (individualist-reformist), and the transformational view (socialist-collectivist). First, the therapeutic view is a foundational idea of social work and it is this view of social work that is dominant in the social work health literature. It conceives of social work as pursuing and engaging in the wellbeing of individuals, groups, and communities by promoting and facilitating growth and self-fulfillment (Payne, 2006). This view focuses on the dynamic interaction that takes place between social workers and their clients.

Second, the social order view sees social work as an element of welfare services for individuals within society (Payne, 2006). Here, social workers adopt maintenance approaches in order to assist people during periods of difficulties until such a time that a state of stability is achieved. According to this view, the aim of social work is to 'solve people's problems in society, by providing help or services' (Payne, 2006, p. 14)—and in that way 'they will fit in with general social expectations better' (p. 14).

Third, the transformational view of social work emphasizes that transformation of societies is required in order for those oppressed to benefit in any significant manner. Here social work strives for more egalitarian relationships in society in order to target disparities of power. In this view, social work embraces the value of equity and believes that individuals cannot achieve personal or social empowerment until large-scale transformations take place. The transformational view asserts that social workers must then 'identify and work out how social relations cause people's problems, and make social changes so that the problems do not arise' (Payne, 2006, p. 14). All three views of social work are important for health.

Apart from providing us with a conceptual framework of social work's three-way discourse, Payne's typology also helps to situate social work within the broader context of health discourses. The typology of social work is a pedagogical tool that can help us to critically assess how compatible approaches to health are with social work values. Further, Payne's (2005, 2006) typology offers students and practitioners a reflexive tool that can be charted to produce a visual representation of where one's own social work discourse falls.

Shaping Curriculum

There are five areas of analysis that are recommended for inclusion in this pedagogical model. The first area is the examination of historical and social processes that have led to the emergence and flourishing of dominant health paradigms. Health and healing always take place within a particular social and historical context (Wright, 2000). This pedagogical model includes an examination of the social and historical factors that have prompted the emergence of dominant health paradigms. This enables students to critically interrogate the reasoning behind the materialization of dominant health paradigms. Knowledge of social and historical factors can provide students with a greater understanding of macro forces and can strengthen a social worker's ability to make decisions about what intervention strategies to employ (Dichter and Cnaan, 2010).

The second component in this pedagogical model is the analysis of the underlying epistemologies that inform the various health paradigms: 'An essential part of critical thinking is the consideration of alternate views ... This aspect of critical thinking involves the appropriate consideration of alternative positions when developing and articulating one's own view or theory' (Bailin and Battersby, 2009, p. 190). The ability to consider alternate positions starts with an exploration of epistemology. Epistemology as a philosophical domain explores not only what constitutes knowledge, but also how knowledge is acquired and produced; what is accepted as truth; and how truth is accepted as such. Epistemology guides discourses, theories and approaches. Maynard (as cited in Crotty, 1998) tells us that 'epistemology is concerned with providing a philosophical grounding for deciding what kinds of knowledge are possible and how we can ensure that they are both adequate and legitimate' (p. 8). Thus, the inclusion of epistemology within the pedagogical model highlights the underlying values and beliefs that shape and guide approaches to health, thus encouraging social workers to consider how foundational values and beliefs assist or negate strategies for overall health and wellbeing. The use of epistemology as a component of the pedagogical model provides an analytic lens through which students can recognize, explore, and evaluate what is promoted as knowledge—including beliefs and values—within a given health paradigm.

The third area for critical exploration is the assumptions about health. Curriculum that is designed around this pedagogical model takes knowledge that is gained from looking at the historical evolution, contributing social processes, and underlying epistemologies to then evaluating what this all means in terms of the assumptions that are made about health and wellness in theory, policy and direct practice. Exploring the assumptions of health that emerge in the various paradigms enables students to assess whether health is understood as an individual or a collective phenomenon. Further, the assumptions of health explores contexts, persons who are involved (often from a differing perspective), related institutional structures, and exposes them to the diversity of language embedded within health. Further, students can then compare and contrast the assumptions about health to determine what strategies best promote and enhance health and wellbeing in relation to social work values.

The fourth component of this model is to critically examine the social work discourse when shaped by a particular health paradigm. Using Payne's (2005, 2006) typology of social work reveals a great deal about how practice can be informed and varied when shaped by differing health perspectives. The use of Payne's (2005, 2006) typology can help with this endeavor by outlining the extent to which social work practice attends to the therapeutic, social order, and transformational views of social work. The exact position of social work practice between these three views may depend on the organizational setting, demands, environment, and individual intervention strategies employed in a given context. However, an approximate position can be identified knowing that this too is not static and dependent on some of the identified factors above. The use of Payne's typography will be illustrated in the next section that introduces six influential health paradigms.

Lastly, the pedagogical model will include a critical examination of how conducive the health paradigms are with social work's values. For example, this will enable students to determine the extent to which approaches within a given health paradigm are consistent with the value of social justice. Social justice is the pursuit of equity in society and is 'concerned with human well-being' (Powers and Faden, 2006, p. 15). As Payne (2005) points out, it is one of the profession's core values. In the examination of health paradigms, coherence with social justice means that we will need to examine the larger systemic and structural forces impacting on health, while constantly recognizing that 'inequalities are interactive' (Powers and Faden, 2006, p. 5). In a recent World Health Organization report, Friedli (2009) describes a need for the inclusion of social justice in approaches to health: 'a focus on social justice may provide an important corrective to what has been seen as a growing over-emphasis on individual pathology' (p. iv). Thus, a critical pedagogical model that explores influential health paradigms can assist social workers to determine how to ground practice in social justice which 'attempt[s] to address immediate crisis and emotional pain while keeping in mind the bigger picture of oppressive policies, practice and social relations' (Baines, 2007, p. 5). This model will challenge students to critically reflect upon strategies that they might employ in practice in a way that is consistent with social work values. The aim is to increase confidence and provide students with a foundation of critical assessment and reflection skills to determine the most appropriate forms of action and approaches.

Influential Health Paradigms

A desire to better understand how health is understood and approached led me to an in-depth academic exploration of the dominant health paradigms shaping discourses. The six most influential paradigms shaping the health discourse include: biomedical, public health, biopsychosocial, social determinants of health, political economy, and holism.

It is recommended at this time that the pedagogical model be structured around these six influential health paradigms; however, this model is intended to be adaptable and fluid. The recommended six paradigms emerged as the most influential health paradigms at the time of this author's research of the literature. Over time, these paradigms may shift or there may be the emergence of a new health paradigm not currently represented in the literature. Thus, omission here of other paradigms is not a statement of their importance or value. It is intended that those who are directly designing their curriculum take into consideration the most influential health paradigms for their locale and time in history. Although these six health paradigms are recommended for inclusion because of the influences that they currently exert in the health discourse, the model can be malleable to include the more dominant paradigms of any given community. My intent here is not to privilege one health paradigm over another, but to suggest that social workers will be better prepared for the realities of practice within the complex system of health by having a foundational understanding of the differences that they will undoubtedly encounter. This knowledge will assist to prepare social workers to take action in the pursuit of health and wellness. What follows is a brief overview of the six influential health paradigms. The intent is not to give a thorough and in-depth review of all aspects of the health paradigms; however, the intent is to illustrate that there are differences amongst the health paradigms and using Payne's (2005, 2006) typography will highlight how these differences can impact on social work discourse.

Biomedical

The most pervasive of health paradigms is biomedicine: it is the current centerpiece of contemporary Western medicine (Longino and Murphy, 1995) and it is 'the dominant paradigm among health care workers and researchers' (Raphael, 2006, p. 126). The biomedical paradigm is firmly rooted in objectivism and embraces reason, objectivity, and moral neutrality. The assumptions of health are focused on health and assume a binary view of health and illness.

The view of social work that emerges when shaped by the biomedical paradigm is illustrated using Payne's (2005, 2006) typology (Figure 1). The view of health promoted by the biomedical paradigm appears to situate social work between the therapeutic view and the social order view of Payne's (2006) three-way discourse. The exact position of social work practice between these two views may depend on the organizational setting, demands, environment, and individual intervention strategies

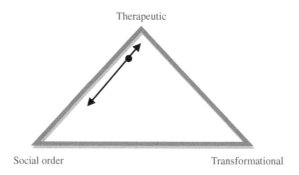

Figure 1 Biomedical Paradigm View of Social Work.

employed in a given context. However, social work practice that equally encompasses the therapeutic and social order views will likely focus on providing services in a dyadic or similarly comprised clinical helping relationship with the emphasis on improving the individual client's capacity for self-sufficiency. The social order view means that social work practice meets individual needs in order for a hospital or medical facility to operate more effectively.

Public Health

Like the biomedical paradigm, the public health paradigm is pervasive in influencing contemporary health and is historically rooted in the West. The public health paradigm is informed by a combination of objectivism and constructionism. Societal links between cause and effect are sought which lead to the development of risk categories and the identification of target populations.

According to Payne's (2005, 2006) typology, social work practice in health as promoted by the public health paradigm appears to fall between the therapeutic and social order view, with some influence of the transformational view (Figure 2). In contrast to the biomedical paradigm, the public health paradigm situates social work practice even closer to both the social order view and to the transformational view.

Social work has been historically linked with the public health paradigm since the 1920s, when the profession expanded to meet the needs of public health's burgeoning preventative programs (Doucet *et al.*, 2001). According to the view of health promoted by the paradigm, social workers are situated among other multidisciplinary professionals as the experts in determining and carrying out intervention strategies. Social work practice revolves around the targets and risk groups identified by epidemiology (Ruth *et al.*, 2008).

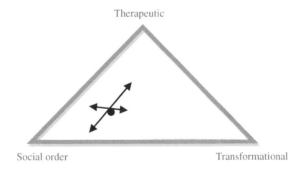

Figure 2 Public Health Paradigm View of Social Work.

Biopsychosocial

The biopsychosocial paradigm has long informed social work curriculum and discourses and is the primary paradigm guiding rehabilitation professionals. The biopsychosocial paradigm assumes a view of health that combines elements of the biomedical paradigm with a social view on health. Thus, health is considered to be

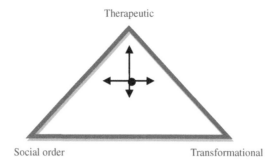

Figure 3 Biopsychosocial Paradigm View of Social Work.

influenced by a combination of physical, psychosocial, and environmental influences. The biopsychosocial paradigm is informed by both objectivism and constructionism whereby knowledge is considered to be both a scientific construct as well as a cultural phenomenon (Stein, 2005).

The biopsychosocial paradigm appears to situate social work closest to the therapeutic view of Payne's typology (2005, 2006) while suggesting some influence from the social order and transformational views (Figure 3). While attending to health needs from the perspective of the biopsychosocial paradigm can occur at both the individual and population level, individual intervention appears to be the most dominant mode of practice for social work. This would situate the social work role at the individual therapeutic view of Payne's typology. A social worker in this role may work independently or may work with any number of health professionals.

The role of social work in the biopsychosocial paradigm also incorporates an element of the transformational view. The individual's environmental context is important and a social worker would likely take into account various structural issues and social processes that impede on one's ability to fully engage in society. Interventions may occur at the 'organizational and/or systems level rather than at an individual level in order to address group-dependent constraints causing disability' (Saleeby, 2007, p. 229). The transformational view may include strategies that include challenging 'social norms, and discriminatory practices that hinder individuals with disabilities, promoting policies and legislation that address the rights of individuals with disabilities, and increasing social supports for individuals with disabilities' (Saleeby, 2007, p. 229).

Social Determinants of Health

The social determinants of health paradigm makes a link between health and various social, environmental, and economic conditions. This paradigm offers 'a window into both the micro-level processes by which social structures lead to individual health or illness and the macro-level processes by which power relationships and political ideology shape the quality of these structures' (Raphael, 2006, p. 132). Knowledge within the social determinants of health paradigm is informed by objectivism,

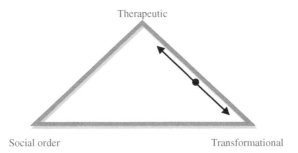

Figure 4   Social Determinants of Health Paradigm View of Social Work.

constructionism, and subjectivism. Social, political, and economic forces are perceived as having the greatest influences on health.

The form of social work practice that transpires from the social determinants of health paradigm is deeply influenced by the transformational view (Figure 4). This paradigm promotes a view of health that requires recognition of, and attendance to, social structures and processes. Because social inequities are the central concern of the social determinants of health paradigm, social work practice under this paradigm views these as a necessary target in order to improve overall health and wellbeing. Social work practice makes overt linkages between health and contextual structures and develops intervention strategies with this in mind; thus, promoting a transformational view of discourse. Social work discourse informed by a social determinants of health paradigm also attends to individual needs by way of the therapeutic view of social work. Health is viewed on an individual and a collective basis.

Political Economy

The political economy paradigm views health as a reaction to a society's political economy and is informed by critical realism. Health is assumed to be a state of physical and emotional wellbeing which includes 'access to and control over the basic material and non material resources that sustain and promote life at a high level of satisfaction' (Baer *et al.*, 1986, p. 95).

Social work practice influenced by the political economy paradigm is associated with the transformational view of Payne's (2005, 2006) typology (Figure 5). This view of social work practice signifies that the focus is committed to the transformation of societies 'for the benefit of the poorest and most oppressed' (p. 13) and practices in a way that views health as a response to social and political factors. From the view of health promoted within the political economy paradigm, the role of social work is to recognize structural influences on health and target policy and structural improvements in practice. To nourish structural change, social work is persuaded to engage in political activity at all levels to influence the creation of more progressive public policy. From a political economy perspective, social work is to be active in recognizing and challenging welfare state structures, as these are considered to be intertwined with the outcomes of health inequalities.

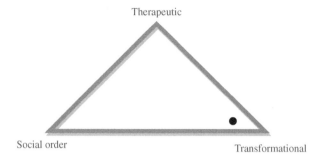

Figure 5 Political Economy Paradigm View of Social Work.

Holism

Two standpoints are located in the holism paradigm: a Western view of holism and a view of health that has been long rooted in indigenous history and traditions (Viergever, 1999; Waldram, 2004). Although both perspectives contain similarities, they each have distinctions that are formed by indigenous epistemology, constructionism and subjectivism. Holism strives for a balance and harmony within the person; health is considered to be one part of a person's entire entity.

Although the view of social work practice that emerges in the holism paradigm may shift when one standpoint is emphasized over another, Payne's (2005, 2006) typology illustrates that all views of social work are fluidly intertwined (Figure 6). Social work practice influenced by the holism paradigm sees that 'any client, be it individual, family, community, is by definition both a part and a whole' (p. 20). This approach influenced by the holism paradigm attends to a variety of variables impacting on a person, interactional and transactional in nature.

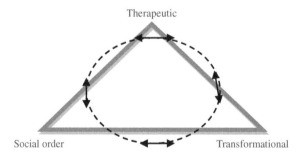

Figure 6 Holism Paradigm View of Social Work.

Conclusion

Shaping curriculum around the dominant health paradigms may seem daunting. However, a minimum of one course that critically exposes social work students to the differences in health will prepare them for practice in a complex system where competing discourses are prevalent. Adequate preparation is important given that social work is actively engaged in the promotion of health and wellbeing. The six dominant paradigms of health have been briefly touched upon to illustrate that there are differences that impact on social work practice. To fully comprehend the dominant health paradigms, a more in-depth critical analysis is needed of the influential historical and social factors, consideration of the driving values and epistemologies, what assumptions are made about health and wellbeing, and the variations in social work roles and strategies based on these larger influences. The knowledge and skills that emerge with the use of this model will challenge students to consider their own views of health and wellbeing. Equally important, this model focuses on developing the most appropriate action and social work response for health and wellbeing.

Shaping curriculum around a pedagogical model that critically assesses dominant health paradigms provides a method of education that is rich in content and thought processes. This approach centralizes conscientization in the educational process; the root of change particularly important in order for one to recognize and have confidence in striving for that change (Freire, 1973; Lavoie, 2001). The use of a deconstruction process as a pedagogical tool fosters critical thinking about larger social and political processes while enabling a sense of critical thought about one's own situation as a social worker. Setting the foundation for social work to develop approaches and strategies that center around health and wellness begins with the adoption of pedagogical models that provide students with the tools and knowledge to critically assess what this means and how to get there.

References

Baer, H., Singer, M. & Johnsen, J. (1986) 'Toward a critical medical anthropology', *Social Science & Medicine*, vol. 34, no. 8, pp. 867–884.

Bailin, S. & Battersby, M. (2009) 'Beyond the boundaries: critical thinking and different cultural perspectives', *Ethics and Education*, vol. 4, no. 2, pp. 189–200.

Baines, D. (2007) 'Anti-oppressive social work practice: fighting for space, fighting for change', in *Doing Anti-Oppressive Practice: Building Transformative Politicized Social Work*, ed. D. Baines, Fernwood, Halifax, pp. 1–30.

Brown, P. (1998) *Understanding and Applying Medical Anthropology*, Mayfield Publishing Company, Mountain View.

Commers, M. (2002) *Determinants of Health: Theory, Understanding, Portrayal, Policy*, Kluwer Academic Publishers, Dordrecht.

Crotty, M. (1998) *The Foundations of Social Research: Meaning and Perspective in the Research Process*, Sage, Thousand Oaks, CA.

Dewees, M. & Lax, L. (2008) 'A critical approach to pedagogy in mental health', *Social Work in Mental Health*, vol. 7, pp. 82–101.

Dichter, M. & Cnaan, R. (2010) 'The benefits of learning social welfare: lessons from student perspectives', *Journal of Teaching in Social Work*, vol. 30, pp. 210–224.

Doucet H., Larouche J. & Melchin K. (eds) (2001) *Ethical Deliberation in Multiprofessional Health Care Teams*, University of Ottawa Press, Ottawa.

Freire, P. (1973) *Education for Critical Consciousness*, Continuum, New York.

Friedli, L. (2009) *Mental Health, Resilience and Inequalities*, World Health Organization, Geneva.

Guba, E. & Lincoln, Y. (2005) 'Paradigmatic controversies, contradictions, and emerging confluences', in *The Sage Handbook of Qualitative Research, Third Edition*, eds N. Denzin & Y. Lincoln, Sage, Thousand Oaks, CA.

Kuhn, T. (1996) *The Structure of Scientific Revolutions*. 3rd edn. University of Chicago Press, Chicago, IL.

Larson, G. (2008) 'Anti-oppressive practice in mental health', *Journal of Progressive Human Services*, vol. 19, no. 1, pp. 39–54.

Lavoie, T. (2001) *Teaching and Learning in Adult and Higher Education: The Example of Anti-Racism and Anti-Oppression Training for Social Work Field Instructors*, unpublished MSW thesis, University of Manitoba, Winnipeg.

Longino, C. & Murphy, J. (1995) *The Old Age Challenge to the Biomedical Model: Paradigm Strain and Health Policy*, Baywood Publishing Company, Amityville.

McArthur, J. (2010) 'Achieving social justice within and through higher education: the challenge for critical pedagogy', *Teaching in Higher Education*, vol. 15, no. 5, pp. 493–504.

Meadows, D. (1999) *Leverage Points: Places to Intervene in a System*, The Sustainability Institute, Hartland.

Millstein, K. H. (1997) 'The taping project: a method for self-evaluation and "informed consciousness" in racism courses', *Journal of Social Work Education*, vol. 33, no. 3, pp. 1–16.

Nelson, G., Lord, J. & Ochocka, J. (2001) *Shifting the Paradigm in Community Mental Health: Towards Empowerment and Community*, University of Toronto Press, Toronto.

Payne, M. (2005) *Modern Social Work Theory*. 3rd edn. Lyceum Books, Chicago, IL.

Payne, M. (2006) *What is Professional Social Work?*, Lyceum Books, Chicago, IL.

Powers, M. & Faden, R. (2006) *Social Justice: The Moral Foundations of Public Health and Health Policy*, Oxford University Press, New York.

Raphael, D. (2006) 'Social determinants of health: an overview of concepts and issues', in *Staying Alive: Critical Perspectives on Health, Illness, and Health Care*, eds D. Raphael, T. Bryant & M. Rioux, Canadian Scholars' Press, Toronto.

Ruth, B., Sisco, S. & Wyatt, J. (2008) 'Public health and social work: training dual professions for the contemporary workplace', *Public Health Reports*, vol. 123, no. 2, pp. 71–77.

Saleeby, P. (2007) 'Applications of a capability approach to disability and the International Classification of Functioning, Disability and Health (ICF) in social work practice', *Journal of Social Work in Disability & Rehabilitation*, vol. 6, no. 1/2, pp. 217–232.

Skelton, A. (2005) *Understanding Teaching Excellence in Higher Education*, Routledge, New York.

Stein, H. (2005) 'It ain't necessarily so: the many faces of the biopsychosocial model', *Families, Systems, & Health*, vol. 23, no. 4, pp. 440–443.

Viergever, M. (1999) 'Indigenous knowledge: an interpretation of views from indigenous peoples', in *What is Indigenous Knowledge? Voices from the Academy*, eds L. Semali & J. Kincheloe, Falmer Press, New York.

Waldram, J. (2004) *Revenge of the Windigo. The Construction of the Mind and Mental Health of North American Aboriginal Peoples*, University of Toronto Press, Toronto.

World Health Organization (WHO) (1992) *World Health Organization: Basic Documents*. 39th edn. World Health Organization, Geneva.

Wright, M. (2000) 'A critical-holistic paradigm for an interdependent world', *American Behavioral Scientist*, vol. 43, no. 5, pp. 808–824.

Teaching Trauma: Critically Engaging a Troublesome Term

Jay Marlowe & Carole Adamson

How the social work profession supports people to live through experiences of trauma and helps to facilitate recovery represents an important base of our practice. Whilst the impacts of trauma in people's lives cannot be discounted, there remains significant scope to further inquire into how people respond to traumatic situations and locate their own sources of healing, hope and survival. Drawing on two different case studies—one with resettled Sudanese refugees in Australia and another involving critical incident debriefing—this paper looks to address the complex intersections between trauma, well-being and the roles of social work pedagogy and practice.

Introduction: Engaging with Trauma

'Trauma' is a term situated in both medical and psychiatric domains but which has also, often uncontested, spread from professional fields into popular currency (Young, 1995; Furedi, 2004). A knowledge base of trauma within social work education is important because of the nature of our clients' experiences and its impact on social workers and yet its meaning is often utilised uncritically. Whilst the etymology of the term goes back to the Greek word for 'wound', it has accrued powerful discursive understandings in numerous professional fields. Within the academic focus on trauma, a clear definition often eludes the reader. It is almost as if this term is taken as an *a priori* understood concept that escapes the need for definition, and that the locus of inquiry begins only after trauma—whether the focus is upon therapeutic approaches, associated sequelae or documenting people's testimony.

Within social work education, trauma is often defined and subsumed within its impact in fields of practice such as child protection and family violence. We contend that its capture within twentieth century scientific classification systems [for instance, the Diagnostic and Statistical Manual (DSM) of the American Psychiatric Association (APA, 1994)] presents social work education with conceptual and philosophical challenges to align concepts of trauma with notions of strengths, recovery and resilience.

This paper discusses the complexities inherent in the conceptualisation of trauma by means of a brief review of trauma and context, illustrated by two social work research studies from different fields. Key issues for the teaching of trauma in social work education are raised. The paper highlights the need to honour and acknowledge the effects and impacts of trauma in people's lives whilst at the same time remaining mindful of their capacities to respond to difficult situations which highlight pathways to well-being and agency.

Trauma in Context and Curricula

Within social work education and curricula, the concept of trauma is one that pervades a number of core teaching foci: human social development; child protection; loss and grief; community work; mental health; and reflective practices. Such a broad application highlights the need to critically engage this term rather than taking it as an *a priori* understood concept. This conceptualisation requires that social workers both acknowledge and validate experiences of trauma whilst at the same time recognising and working with people's resiliencies, pathways to healing and ability to create meaning in its wake. Social work's focus on systems and broader structural social forces, constructivist orientations and strengths-based tenets provides a helpful orientation to critically engage with bio-medical traditions that often privilege symptomatology over context.

Much of our current understanding and teaching of trauma is predicated upon its description and classification captured within the nosological systems of the DSM and the International Classification of Diseases (ICD) (World Health Organisation, 1992). First mention of trauma in the DSM came with the third edition in 1980: post-traumatic stress disorder (PTSD) was the first classification in this diagnostic manual to explicitly acknowledge external causation (a stressor) of the symptoms of distress (APA, 1980). Putting the context into trauma has, as van der Kolk and McFarlane (1996, p. 4) suggest, enabled the study of trauma to become the 'soul of psychiatry'. They observe that the conceptual development of PTSD has provided the framework for looking at the interconnections between biology, personality and construction of meaning that is dependent upon time and place.

Notwithstanding the admission of the importance of context within the classification of trauma, there remains a tension between the bio-medical and the more ecologically and constructivist-informed constructions of human experience. Acute stress disorder (ASD) was introduced in DSM-IV (APA, 1994) in recognition of a variance in pathways of traumatic response over time. Much of the current debate over the formulation of post-traumatic syndromes in DSM-V (to be published in 2012) has occurred around issues of quantifying and defining the nature of stressors, their pathways into traumatic symptomatology and the philosophical shift associated with the acceptance that traumatisation is as much reliant on context as it is on the original event(s). It is likely that DSM-V will introduce categories of traumatic experience that are more closely positioned in recognition of complex pathways (for instance, in situations of early childhood abuse or multiple exposures to domestic violence or civil war). The exploration of such multiple pathways into and out of traumatic experience opens further opportunity for dialogue with the knowledge bases of social work, whether in child protection, refugee resettlement, mental health, natural disasters or numerous other fields.

Trauma and Social Work Education

The increasing recognition of context in the conceptualisation of trauma provides social work education with the opportunity to introduce scientifically and ecologically informed understandings into the curriculum. It is also our contention that a social work articulation of trauma, informed by environmental and cultural dimensions, can be at the cutting edge of current constructions of trauma: the following case studies serve as an illustration of this.

Considering how the experiences of trauma pervade social work practice, there is relatively scant literature that focuses upon delivering the complexities of a trauma-informed curriculum. There is, however, a growing literature that examines working with post-traumatic stress (Fournier, 2002; Robert, 2002), moving beyond dominant discourses on trauma (McKenzie Mohr, 2004; Bussey, 2008; Breckenridge and James, 2010) and how to work through vicarious traumatisation (Miller, 2001; Cunningham, 2004; Nuttman-Shwartz and Dekel, 2008). Breckenridge and James (2010) provide an example of how a social work curriculum with a focus on trauma can be conceptualised from individual to community-based interventions. Within their course, the term 'therapeutic' moves beyond a simple engagement with therapy to incorporate the concepts of helpfulness, well-being and social justice. This focus moves beyond, but is not discrediting of, bio-medical perspectives. A central tenet of this broader engagement is that the initial impact of trauma (perhaps individual with physical and/or psychological consequences) plays out through transmutation into social and community-level effects over time and space.

The two following case studies, from different fields, serve to illustrate the argument of this paper that a social work construction of a trauma knowledge base can inform a contextually vibrant and critical curriculum. Underpinning both pieces of research was the fundamental issue of needing to recognise how trauma is conceptualised to inform best practices. Blumer (1969) introduces the idea of *sensitising concepts*, which gives the inquirer the initial ideas to pursue a particular topic or research question. The sensitising concepts for both of these projects came from social work practice experience with those living through experiences of loss, extreme stress and trauma. These experiences provided sensitisation to ask particular questions such as how do people respond to, and define, trauma? The research sought to explore what were the pathways to recovery and how people held on to their hopes and dreams despite what they had been through. By recording the narrative accounts of people's experiences, we could seek to understand more fully what informed a person's response(s) to trauma and how they challenged, incorporated and responded to its effects. The two case studies challenged us as social workers to think about best practice with regard to trauma and to critically examine the assumptions about trauma that we brought to the first interpersonal encounter and to understanding the journey of recovery.

The case studies are chosen to illustrate the interaction of trauma and resilience not only in a 'client' group but also within employment environments as both provide helpful perspectives for the development of a trauma curriculum in social work education. The first case study discusses a research project with resettled Sudanese refugees and their perspectives on trauma from forced migration and resettlement contexts; the second examines the issues involved in critical incident debriefing within organisational settings.

Case Study One: Sudanese Refugees Resettling in Australia

The first case study incorporates a three-year research project documenting the in-depth narratives of 24 Sudanese men who had resettled in Adelaide, Australia as former refugees (see Marlowe, 2009, 2010a). The study's focus was to establish how these men, who were fluent in English and often leaders in their community, conceptualise and respond to situations involving trauma. Analysis was carried out through a process of initial and focused coding, writing memos, theoretical sampling and using the constant comparative method as per constructivist grounded theory (Charmaz, 2006). In total, 70 interviews with the 24 participants were conducted.

It was initially thought that participants would need a concise definition of trauma for their reference but it was found to be a term highly familiar to them. It is a word they learned that would help them gain entry into refugee camps, establish claims for refugee status, and qualify for services in Australia. In this respect, trauma represented a form of currency that laid their claims for recognition and access to vital resources (Marlowe, 2010b). It was thus decided to allow participants to express trauma on their own terms and this provided opportunities to better understand how they respond to difficult experiences and what they view as their most salient concerns. Regardless of one's definition of trauma, it would be contentious to claim that the participants' narratives did not embody elements of trauma. However, the *experiences of trauma* and being *a traumatised person* can be very different things.

> We need to get rid of that thinking that our people are traumatised. We were traumatised, yes this is true and that is fine. But that does not mean what we are. We are something different and we can provide. We can offer. We can contribute. (Participant 18)

Whilst there is no question that forced migration can be traumatising, it does not necessarily follow that a refugee is a traumatised person. This perspective is highly important if resettled refugees are to be able to participate as equals in civic society. Echoing Silove and Ekbald's (2002) warning, if refugees are presented to host countries as psychologically traumatised, the debate over asylum can easily move from humanitarian responsibilities and protection to inevitable economic implications and associated public fears of accepting refugees.

In terms of reporting what the men identified as being traumatic, it needs to be emphasised that this research does not challenge the fact that a number of refugees have experienced psychological distress and traumatisation. A number of participants describe the negative experiences associated with forced migration as 'war trauma' and having a 'hangover from the war'. A Sudanese participant elaborates on such hangovers with respect to how the community is coping with such difficult experiences and their perspectives on recovery:

> We are not there yet [recovery] but growing towards that because we still have a *hangover* from the war yet in this area. There is peace but there are remnants of the hangover that caused all that to happen, which are still, you know, creeping up. They are still surfacing. (Participant 8)

It is critical that social workers acknowledge these 'hangovers' as such experiences can have very real negative impacts on people's physical and mental well-being. Most participants, however, were quick to emphasise that political violence and war-related trauma do not necessarily embody an indelibly deleterious impact. In fact, there were numerous ways that participants were able to respond to these difficulties; responses that situate the participants as active agents who have skills and knowledge to use towards healing, coping and recovery.

Though all participants spoke of the trauma associated with forced migration, many noted that adapting to the new social realities in a new host country was as difficult (if not more so) than the adversities associated with forced migration. Such comments reinforce the importance of understanding their challenges holistically and how people create meaning within new social, political and cultural landscapes. As Westoby (2006, p. 157) writes about Sudanese people's lives within the contested landscapes of trauma and recovery, 'There is little space for refugee voices to interrupt these colonizing processes and articulate their own aspirations for reconstructing a social world that would facilitate well-being on their terms'. Part of promoting well-being on participants' terms is allowing them to express their conceptualisations of, and responses to, trauma rather than making *a priori* assumptions about it.

Overall, participants were critical of what they called 'Western' counselling approaches that focussed on talking about trauma in an unfamiliar agency setting. Rather, they spoke about the importance of establishing a relationship with the community (often within the community as opposed to within an agency) and how professionals could play an integral role in working alongside them to greater realise practical outcomes related to employment, education and suitable housing. These findings are not suggesting that negative mental health outcomes are not possibly present or that Western-based psychosocial interventions are not needed. Rather, it is after issues such as affordable housing, access to employment, English language acquisition and educational training are addressed (often situated in structural considerations) that the interpersonal work of resolving psychopathological sequelae can be better addressed, if resonant and needed.

This study highlighted that the Sudanese community has numerous pathways for responding to trauma, which reinforce diverse individual and community knowledges about healing and recovery. It follows that participants responded to trauma through the important social and cultural functions located within the community milieu. Others identified the role of spirituality and agential realisations of employment and education as pathways that embodied hope and offered resonant responses to trauma. Importantly, participants also identified that social work professionals can also play integral roles in working towards resettling community's hopes and aspirations. Participants repeatedly noted how, in resettlement contexts, the hope for a better future has helped them to work through and move beyond traumatic experiences. The array of psychosocial interventions, engaging with structural forces and the practical outcomes of finding employment, pursuing an education and assisting people to navigate the different social realities between home and host countries highlights the multiple social work roles in fostering such hopes.

Case Study Two: Critical Incident Debriefing

In the second case study, the focus of traumatic experience moves from the refugee and resettlement arena to the organisational focus of critical incidents and traumatic events within the New Zealand workplace (Adamson, 2006). The narratives of 20 mental health workers, ranging in professional orientation from psychiatrists, social workers and other professionals through to untrained support workers and those selected on the basis of cultural expertise, were considered in the light of what factors enabled individuals affected by severely stressful experiences to cope with and process the events.

Theoretical analysis of the literature and the narratives was structured by the use of two systemic and holistically informed frameworks: an ecological perspective (Bronfenbrenner, 1979; Harvey, 1996; Harney, 2007) and a uniquely New Zealand model, Te Whare Tapa Wha (Durie, 1994; Rochford, 2004). Both of these models underpin much social work education in New Zealand. The ecological perspective is envisaged as a series of inter-related systems that locate the unique individual within bi-directional influences of the immediate environment alongside societal, cultural and structural factors. Te Whare Tapa Wha has its identity within a Maori world view. Symbolising the necessary four walls of a house, the elements of health in this representation are portrayed as *te taha hinengaro* (mental processes), *te taha tinana* (physical processes), *te taha whanau* (family and social processes) and *te taha wairua* (spiritual processes). Health and well-being are achieved by maintaining a balance in each of these areas. Both frameworks recognise the interconnected, reciprocal and mutually inter-dependent levels of human experience and served within the research as a conceptual platform to critically deconstruct the knowledge bases and impact of traumas. From a social work perspective, these models enable links to be made between individual traumatic experience on physiological, cognitive and behavioural levels and the impact on organisations, communities, societies and human rights.

Research participants were asked to nominate and describe incidents that they deemed to be critical incidents or traumatic events. No attempt was made by the researcher to categorise or diagnose the experiences as either traumatic, a crisis or as highly stressful: participants attested to their own perception of criticality in incidents as diverse as being called 'unprofessional' as a new graduate, to multiple exposures to sudden death, suicide attempts and assaults. Rather, the narratives were considered in the light of trauma concepts from both scientific and holistic perspectives, offering the possibilities of a multi-focused interpretation of experience inclusive of individual understanding and need as well as a contextualised focus on environmental factors in resilience and recovery.

For the majority of participants, the initial events (a suicide, assault or indecent exposure, for instance) were located in the nature of, and roles within, the professional environment. As in the first case study, any narratives were suggestive of the emergence of both the impacts of trauma and people's responses to them. The stressful and potentially damaging physical and emotional reactions experienced by participants were nonetheless balanced in their narratives by accounts of appropriate personal and professional responses such as stemming blood flow from a severed artery or calling for police back-up in a riot. The different levels of experience and interpretation thus offer potentially divergent pathways for recovery.

What proved most affirmative or deleterious to health and well-being, however, was the nature of the subsequent organisational response. In some cases, successful coping with shock and crisis was sabotaged over time by organisational and environmental amnesia or minimisation, or by poorly supported processes related to the worker's involvement in the client's ongoing situation. In others, supportive management and affirmation of professional actions actively engaged with recovery and the re-establishment of personal resilience. In some of the situations that may have resonated with a scientific diagnosis of post-traumatic syndromes, the deep impact (flashbacks, emotional arousal and cognitive–behavioural avoidance) occurred during meaning-making processes in subsequent months after the initial precipitating event, suggesting that the *shape* of the traumatic experience was determined considerably by post-experience response from others in the environment rather than solely by the individual.

Literature concerning social worker responses to highly stressful work environments confirms that the workplace conditions contain both the potential for damage and for growth and healing (for instance, Huxley *et al.*, 2005; Collins, 2008). Support processes (such as structural management responses), systemic factors (such as vertical as well as lateral communication channels and collaborative teamwork), professional practices (such as supervision and individual opportunities for meaning-making) can all encourage resiliency and strengthen what Lindy (1985) termed the 'trauma membrane'.

The debates over critical incident stress debriefing (CISD) and its location within organisational stress-management programmes proved to be a focal point for the discussion of the research findings. Not only did the debate over debriefing have all the hallmarks of ideological tensions between the knowledge bases of bio-medical psychiatry and psychology (Bisson *et al.*, 2000; Deahl, 2000; Kenardy, 2000; Gold and Faust, 2002) and the emergency services personnel from whom critical incident stress debriefing emerged (Everly *et al.*, 2000), but it highlighted the crucial importance of environmental conditions in the experience, impact and interpretation of, and recovery from, critical incidents and traumatic events in the workplace. Emerging out of the debate were key differences in the interpretation of the trauma definition, reliant in some perspectives on the neurological identifiers of brain and behaviour, and promoted in some contexts as synonymous with crisis, emergency and high stress levels.

In addition, participants' narratives from the critical incidents' and traumatic events' research provided a critique of the debriefing debate itself. Whilst the outcome of the debate has strongly recommended the cessation of compulsory debriefing processes and a reduction of emotional content in order to reduce the potential for secondary or re-traumatisation (British Psychological Society, 2002), the focus on trauma and stress symptoms and individual impact overlooks the key operational elements of critical incidents within the workplace. Key to the CISD orthodoxy is the insistence that debriefing is not an operational review (Mitchell, 1995), a statement aimed at avoiding blame-throwing and the power dynamics of responsibility and accountability. However, the mental health workers in this research were committed to professional development and learning from the incidents: questions such as *what can I/we do better?* ranked alongside *how can we improve things for the client/organisation?* Professional practice issues thus emerged as part of the meaning-making process for the participants. Such contextual attention suggests that, in an analysis of the response to traumas, we ignore the environment at our peril.

Discussion: Engaging Trauma in the Curriculum

What can these case studies suggest for social work education? They represent social work research in diverse fields, yet both signal a critical engagement with dominant discourses regarding the discursive understandings of trauma and perspectives on healing and recovery. These studies also illustrate the importance of social work research in the development of a trauma-informed curriculum. We use the term 'curriculum' here to highlight the value of embedding a trauma-informed approach across the many substantive areas of social work education. The experience of living through loss and trauma is one of the few strands that retains salience across the entire social work curriculum; whether it is about mental health, reflective practices, the transgenerational impacts of colonisation, child protection or working with addictions. It is from this perspective that several core principles for social work education emerge from the consideration of these two studies.

First, the case studies illustrate the importance of research-informed teaching that can challenge the anecdotal and popular perception of 'trauma-as-disaster' often taken as fact. Incorporating rigour into our research and teaching can help traverse the discursive territories of trauma to think not only about its impacts but also about people's capacities to recover. Whilst the case studies illustrate the human capacity for resilience and growth, this focus can often be overshadowed by our strong reactions to horrendous experience(s). Both studies suggest that work with any groups or individuals affected by what is broadly termed trauma or crisis is required to be conducted in a considered manner that goes beyond the common monikers of the 'refugee experience' and 'getting over it' and attempts to comprehend the discursive constructions of the experience for those involved. It means turning the mirror on ourselves and our practice so that it is possible to critically examine our own assumptions, training and ways of working with people living through loss, extreme stress and trauma. These comments reinforce Freire's (1990) assertion that social workers need to embrace a 'critical curiosity' whereby we are curious, not only about the lives and actions of those that we work alongside, but also about our own. Incorporating sensitising concepts into our teaching and facilitating students to think critically about their assumptions and how these may influence social work encounters is, we argue, an imperative for social work education.

Secondly, the social work curriculum must critically engage with concepts of trauma to recognise the tensions between (and values of) bio-medical and alternative perspectives. This focus requires incorporating the associated cultural, biological and historical dimensions of trauma. As Kirmayer (2007, p. 4) states:

> Like any generative trope, the metaphor of trauma shapes our thinking in ways that are both explicit and hidden. The history of trauma, then, is not simply a story of the march of scientific, medical, and psychiatric progress toward greater clarity about a concept with fixed meaning, but a matter of changing social constructions of experience, in the context of particular clinical, cultural and political ideologies.

It is necessary to acknowledge that bio-medical perspectives provide important insights into increased risk factors for both physical and mental health well-being. Alternative perspectives that incorporate a broader or more holistic purview to people's lives are also needed. The recognition that people are capable of making meaningful and lasting responses to trauma which situate them beyond a simple victimised or damaged perspective is essential if promoting health and well-being— with clients or with colleagues—is to be a foundation of our work. This multi-focused approach to trauma helps practitioners, researchers, educators and students to recognise the potentially deleterious impacts of trauma while also acknowledging that there is not a causal pathway to such outcomes. This shifted focus from traumatised individuals to asking why particularly difficult experiences have occurred can also help to render other important considerations visible that include: structural inequalities; unjust social policies; and the domains of power. These broader levels can directly impact upon local forms of healing, resistance and recovery from traumatic experiences.

Third, whilst acknowledging that some people experience ongoing adverse mental health outcomes from traumatic events, the resilience literature also provides important reminders that many do not suffer from long-term psychological problems or are indelibly damaged people (Calhoun and Tedeschi, 2000; Updegraff and Taylor, 2000). This suggests an incorporation of theories of resilience and a strengths approach to working with trauma within the social work curriculum. The participant comments also demonstrate that the experience of potentially traumatising events is best understood from within the narratives of those thus exposed. It further reinforces that the comprehension of the experience and the associated social work interventions must acknowledge and dignify the trauma story whilst at the same time look for stories of agency, hope and survival.

Finally, the participants in these two pieces of research have an important message for the manner in which social work education can reinforce effectiveness in our work. Both the dislocations of the refugee experience and those of the organisationally-based critical incidents were only the beginnings of the experiences that can be uncritically labelled as 'traumatic'. Both groups witnessed that, in many cases, the most challenging experiences were not the initial events, but the playing out of the experience over time. The interplay of context and response (rather than events themselves) proved the most testing to resilience and hope. The social work role, in all its manifestations of structural assistance, community building, systems negotiation as well as in validation of narratives, is a crucial but under-recognised trauma activity. It means recognising that the present influences the past and that the level of our analysis must go beyond traumas predicated in the past. The experience of trauma is embedded in a process which necessitates an examination of the present. We are suggesting that the holistic incorporation of a person's embedded experience across multiple levels (which include time and place) offers a solid framework for addressing the conceptual challenges of engaging with trauma in our profession's numerous substantive fields.

These two case studies provide some helpful direction in the consideration of trauma within the social work curriculum. They suggest that whilst there is merit in addressing 'trauma' as a specific topic, there is much to be gained from unpacking its meaning and highlighting the many and various interconnections with established social work processes and interventions. The voices of the participants teach us that sensitisation to the relationship of the ordinary (the necessities of daily life, environmental supports, a sense of identity and belonging) to the extreme (the catastrophe, the dislocations, the initial experiences of 'traumas') is crucial in honouring their stories of recovery and hope.

Conclusion

Maintaining a critical and evidence-based approach to trauma represents an important cornerstone of the social work profession and education. It means locating the discursive perspectives and power domains of related practice in which social workers find themselves inextricably entwined. There is a powerful need to honour, validate and dignify the impacts and experiences of trauma. There is also an imperative for remembering that such experiences are not identity statements or automatic pathways to deleterious outcomes and that, for social work and social work education, responses and interventions may be trauma-informed but not necessarily trauma-focused. If trauma, as Furedi (2004) maintains, has colonised both the professional and the every day, social work has an important role to engage this term critically and holistically within the many substantive fields of our practice.

Acknowledgements

We would like to thank Tricia Bingham for her assistance in the library and Sue Osborne for providing editorial advice.

References

Adamson, C. (2006) *Complexity and Context: Staff Support Systems in Mental Health After Critical Incidents and Traumatic Events.* Unpublished Doctoral Thesis, Massey University, Wellington, New Zealand.

American Psychiatric Association (APA) (1980) *Diagnostic and Statistical Manual of Mental Disorders.* 3rd edn. American Psychiatric Association, Washington, DC.

American Psychiatric Association (APA) (1994) *Diagnostic and Statistical Manual of Mental Disorders.* 4th edn. American Psychiatric Association, Washington, DC.

Bisson, J. I., McFarlane, A. C. & Rose, S. (2000) 'Psychological debriefing', in *Effective Treatments for PTSD: Practice Guidelines from the International Society for Traumatic Stress Studies*, eds T. M. Keane, M. J. Freidman & E. B. Foa, Guilford, New York, pp. 39–59.

Blumer, H. (1969) *Symbolic Interactionism*, Prentice-Hall, Engle-Wood Cliffs, NJ.

Breckenridge, J. & James, K. (2010) 'Educating social work students in multifaceted interventions for trauma', *Social Work Education*, vol. 29, no. 3, pp. 259–275.

British Psychological Society (Professional Practice Board Working Party) (2002) *Psychological Debriefing*, Leicester [online]. Available at: http://www.bps.org.uk.

Bronfenbrenner, U. (1979) *The Ecology of Human Development*, Harvard University Press, Cambridge, MA.

Bussey, M. C. (2008) 'Trauma response and recovery certificate program: preparing students for effective practice', *Journal of Teaching in Social Work*, vol. 28, no. 1/2, pp. 117–144.

Calhoun, L. G. & Tedeschi, R. G. (2000) 'Early post-traumatic interventions: facilitating possibilities for growth', in *Posttraumatic Stress Intervention: Challenges, Issues & Perspectives*, eds D. Paton, C. Dunning, J. M. Violanti & Charles C. Thomas, Springfield, IL, pp. 135–152.

Charmaz, K. (2006) *Constructing Grounded Theory*, Sage Publications, London.

Collins, S. (2008) 'Statutory social workers: stress, job satisfaction, coping, social support and individual differences', *British Journal of Social Work*, vol. 38, no. 6, pp. 1173–1193.

Cunningham, M. (2004) 'Teaching social workers about trauma: reducing the risks of vicarious traumatization in the classroom', *Journal of Social Work Education*, vol. 40, no. 2, pp. 305–317.

Deahl, M. (2000) 'Psychological debriefing: controversy and challenge', *Australian and New Zealand Journal of Psychiatry*, vol. 34, no. 6, pp. 929–939.

Durie, M. (1994) *Whaiora: Maori Health Development*, Oxford University Press, Auckland.

Everly, G. S., Flannery, R. B. & Mitchell, J. T. (2000) 'Critical incident stress management (CISM): a review of the literature', *Aggression and Violent Behavior*, vol. 5, no. 1, pp. 23–40.

Fournier, R. (2002) 'A trauma education workshop for posttraumatic stress', *Health & Social Work*, vol. 27, no. 2, pp. 113–124.

Freire, P. (1990) 'A critical understanding of social work', *Journal of Progressive Human Services*, vol. 1, no. 1, pp. 3–9.

Furedi, F. (2004) *Therapy Culture: Cultivating Vulnerability in an Uncertain Age*, Routledge, London.

Gold, S. N. & Faust, J. (2002) 'The future of trauma practice: visions and aspirations', *Journal of Trauma Practice*, vol. 1, no. 1, pp. 1–15.

Harney, P. A. (2007) 'Resilience processes in context: contributions and implications of Bronfenbrenner's person–process–context model', *Journal of Aggression, Maltreatment and Trauma*, vol. 14, no. 3, pp. 73–87.

Harvey, M. R. (1996) 'An ecological view of psychological trauma and trauma recovery', *Journal of Traumatic Stress*, vol. 9, no. 1, pp. 3–23.

Huxley, P., Evans, S., Gately, C., Webber, M., Mears, A., Pajak, S., Kendall, T., Medina, J. & Katona, C. (2005) 'Stress and pressures in mental health social work: the worker speaks', *British Journal of Social Work*, vol. 35, no. 7, pp. 1063–1079.

Kenardy, J. (2000) 'The current status of psychological debriefing', *British Medical Journal*, vol. 321, 28 October, pp. 1032–1033.

Kirmayer, L. (2007) 'Failures of imagination: the refugee's predicament', in *Understanding Trauma: Integrating Biological, Clinical, and Cultural Perspectives*, eds L. Kirmayer, R. Lemelson & M. Barad, Cambridge University Press, New York.

Lindy, J. (1985) 'The trauma membrane and other clinical concepts derived from psychotherapeutic work with survivors of natural disasters', *Psychiatric Annals*, vol. 15, pp. 153–160.

Marlowe, J. (2009) 'Accessing authentic knowledge: being and doing with the Sudanese community', *Australian Community Psychologist*, vol. 21, no. 1, pp. 39–49.

Marlowe, J. (2010a) 'Using a narrative approach of double listening in research contexts', *The International Journal of Narrative Therapy and Community Work*, no. 3, pp. 43–53.

Marlowe, J. (2010b) 'Beyond the discourse of trauma: shifting the focus on Sudanese refugees', *Journal of Refugee Studies*, vol. 23, no. 2, pp. 183–198.

McKenzie Mohr, S. (2004) 'Creating space for radical trauma theory in generalist social work education', *Journal of Progressive Human Services*, vol. 15, no. 2, pp. 45–55.

Miller, M. (2001) 'Creating a safe frame for learning: teaching about trauma and trauma treatment', *Journal of Teaching in Social Work*, vol. 21, no. 3/4, pp. 159–176.

Mitchell, J. T. (1995) 'Essentials of critical incident stress management', in *Innovations in Disaster and Trauma Psychology, Volume One: Applications in Emergency Services and Disaster Response*, ed. G. S. Everly, Chevron, Ellicott City, MD, pp. 68–89.

Nuttman-Shwartz, O. & Dekel, R. (2008) 'Training students for a shared traumatic reality', *Social Work*, vol. 53, no. 3, pp. 279–281.

Robert, R. (2002) 'A trauma education workshop on posttraumatic stress', *Health & Social Work*, vol. 27, no. 2, pp. 113–124.

Rochford, T. (2004) 'Whare tapa wha: a Māori model of a unified theory of health', *The Journal of Primary Prevention*, vol. 25, no. 1, pp. 41–57.

Silove, D. & Ekblad, S. (2002) 'How well do refugees adapt after resettlement in Western countries?', *Acta Psychiatrica Scandinavica*, vol. 106, no. 6, pp. 401–402.

Updegraff, J. & Taylor, S. E. (2000) 'From vulnerability to growth: positive and negative effects of stressful life events', in *Loss and Trauma: General and Close Relationship Perspectives*, eds J. H. Harvey & E. H. Miller, Brunner-Routledge, Philadelphia, PA, pp. 3–28.

van der Kolk, B. A. & McFarlane, A. C. (1996) 'The black hole of trauma', in *Traumatic Stress: The Effects of Overwhelming Experience on Mind, Body and Society*, eds B. A. van der Kolk, A. C. McFarlane & L. Weisaeth, The Guilford Press, New York, pp. 3–23.

Westoby, P. (2006) *The Sociality of Healing Engaging Southern Sudanese Refugees Resettling in an Australian Context: A Model of Social Healing*. Doctoral Thesis, University of Queensland, Australia.

World Health Organisation (WHO) (1992) *ICD-10: International Statistical Classification of Diseases and Related Health Problems*, 10th revision, World Health Organisation, Geneva.

Young, A. (1995) *The Harmony of Illusions: Inventing Post Traumatic Stress Disorder*, Princeton University Press, Princeton, NJ.

Developing Wellbeing as a Critical Tool in Social Work Education: An Example from the Field of Learning Disability

Graeme Simpson

This paper will explore how 'wellbeing' is used in social work education to develop a critical understanding of the current English personalisation agenda, in relation to people with 'moderate to severe' learning disabilities. Drawing upon a short thematic analysis of policy for Learning Disability and Social Work Education, the paper will develop the argument that social wellbeing is an important factor for critical engagement and practice with this service-user group. Based upon teaching – incorporating service user and care views, as well as current research-in-progress, Schalock's (2004) taxonomy of wellbeing is developed to focus upon three themes: friendships and relationships; community engagement and structural factors. The importance for social workers of exploring aspects of community, in its widest sense, is emphasised, contrasting with a narrower view presented in policy implementation. The application of wellbeing as a practice and analytical concept therefore provides a framework for a critically reflective and engaged practice.

Introduction

The paper explores the use of 'wellbeing' in social work education, in relation to practitioners and students in the field of adult learning disability. First, the policy framework for people with a learning disability in England[1] is established and briefly analysed through a discussion of 'normalisation' and the 'social model of disability'. There follows a brief thematic analysis of these policies and also those of social work education, identifying the relative absence of wellbeing. Though Dominelli and Hackett (2010, p. 755) regard wellbeing as a 'slippery concept', the World Health

Organisation (1986, p. 1) promoted a definition of 'social wellbeing' emphasising 'social and personal resources'. The paper develops arguments for including wellbeing in social work education, followed by examples of how this can be achieved, based upon experiences of short courses at Masters and Post-Qualifying level in England, but with reference to other countries to establish the global nature of its application. The final section of the paper examines aspects of the educational programme in more detail and draws upon research-in-progress with people with learning disabilities, establishing how wellbeing can be used to promote critical reflection and engagement.

Policy Framework for People with Learning Disability

Valuing People (DOH, 2001) was a document outlining the UK government's policy for this group of service users. Its progress has been charted through government papers, most recently, *Valuing People Now* (DOH, 2008). The policy draws from two paradigms: 'normalisation' and the 'social model of disability', both of which originated in an analysis of previous policies towards people with learning disabilities.

In the mid-nineteenth century institutions were places of safety for people with learning disabilities, who were 'rescued' from abusing families (Ryan with Thomas, 1987). This developed into a policy of segregating people with learning disabilities from the rest of society, underscored by social Darwinism (Oliver, 1990; Race, 2007). At its extreme, it resulted in the incarceration of people with learning disabilities— frequently against their will and that of their family (Rolph *et al.*, 2005)—perfecting capitalist society's need for a mechanism of social control (Foucault, 1979). This was not confined to England, with similar developments charted in Australia (Bigby and Atkinson, 2010) and in a German context by Knust-Potter (1998). Many families kept their children at home (Rolph *et al.*, 2003; Hreinsdottir *et al.*, 2006), yet people with learning disabilities experienced social exclusion, whether segregated in an institution, or 'hidden' within the family. In response, Nirje (1969), in Sweden, and Wolfensberger (1972), in Canada, developed the concept of 'normalisation', later taken up by self-advocacy groups from the late 1960s and 1970s onwards (Flynn and Lemay, 1999).

Normalisation cannot be seen as a 'unified' model and Shakespeare (2006, p. 22) identifies two developmental strands. Nirje's (1969, p. 19) 'Scandinavian' approach was premised upon 'rights', whereas Wolfensberger's approach emphasised the *social devaluation* of this group, across most developed welfare regimes (Race, 2003). Despite the different emphasis, the outcomes were quite similar: both sought to ensure that the 'conditions of everyday life [for people with learning disabilities] ... are as close as possible to the norms and patterns of the mainstream of society' (Nirje, 1969, p. 19).

One criticism is that this approach implies an accommodation with the mainstream potentially resulting in policies which not only 'de-institutionalise', but also implies that people with learning disabilities should not associate with one another and seek out 'normal' friends (Shakespeare, 2006, p. 22). A further critique is that much of the normalisation research was undertaken by the 'able-bodied', though this is perhaps understandable given the level of intellectual disability (Shakespeare, 2006, p. 23). Within *Valuing People* (DOH, 2001, 2008) normalisation is seen as progressive, but it is based upon a romanticism of the policy, which sees the most able as representative of the whole group (Burton and Kagan, 2006).

The social model of disability, another influence on policy development, has frequently criticised 'normalisation'. Oliver (2001), in his materialist critique, argues that 'normalisation' is based upon functionalist sociology and offers 'no satisfactory explanation of *why* disabled people are oppressed in capitalist societies and no strategy for liberating us from the chains of that oppression' (Oliver, 2001, p. 4). For Oliver, people with learning disabilities need to have their situation understood in a materialist way, through understanding the nature of capitalist society. He argues that the difficulties people with learning disabilities face 'cannot be described solely in terms of the normality/abnormality dichotomy and inegalitarian social structures cannot be explained by reference only to valued and devalued social roles' (Oliver, 2001, p. 8).

There is a significant difference in the two models of disability, notably in their theoretical development and construction. Race *et al.* (2005) acknowledge these differences, but claim these are often overstated in the academic debates, arguing for a 'dialogue for practice' to counter the oppressions, which people with learning disabilities face daily (2005, p. 519). Thus, there is a move towards a debate which focuses upon policy and practice.

Acknowledging the influence of competing paradigms, the role of wellbeing within the policy will now be analysed. The focus upon social inclusion through work, community participation and choice (Burton and Kagan, 2006; Simpson and Price, 2010), appears to promote elements of wellbeing. Yet, within the document *Valuing People*, 'wellbeing' is only specifically referred to twice: first, in relation to wider 'strategies for improving access to education, housing and employment which enhance and promote mental wellbeing [and which] will include people with learning disabilities and mental health problems' (DOH, 2001, s6.25, p. 66); second, in regard to local strategic partnerships, which aim 'to simplify and expand the scope of partnerships concerned with community wellbeing' (DOH, 2001, s9, p. 107). In *Valuing People Now* (DOH, 2008) there are no specific references to wellbeing. Both documents, however, discuss the complex health, housing and employment needs, which contribute to 'wellbeing' but which are subservient to the over-riding concept of 'choice'.

If 'quality of life', as opposed to 'wellbeing' was identified there is little to add. The first two references are to an improved quality of life through de-institutionalisation (DOH, 2001, pp. 16 and 75) and the only other reference is to improved leisure opportunities (DOH, 2001, p. 80). *Valuing People Now* only refers to:

> Services across transport, leisure, education, health, housing, community safety and the criminal justice system and access to information and advice are vital to ensuring people's independence and overall quality of life. (DOH, 2008, p. 7)

Valuing People is not the only government policy which shapes practice in this field. *Personalisation* is often used as a 'catch-all' term for the trend to devolve budgets to individuals, who then make choices as to how they spend this money, and thus is arguably of greater significance. Such policies have long been advocated by many disability rights groups and have been championed by the *In Control* group (Duffy, 2010). For people with learning disabilities, Burton and Kagan (2006, p. 305) suggest this summarises a utopia which:

> sees people making choices about activities in pleasant neighbourhoods, with plentiful community resources. They are supported in this by their own staff, which they employ, and who work to their specification. They are likely to be in work, and to have friendships and relationships, mostly with non-disabled people.

Thereby the difficulties in ensuring that people with learning disabilities receive proper support are 'glossed over' as 'an inadvertent trick takes place where the least impaired people are used in the imagery to stand for all the others' (Burton and Kagan, 2006, p. 306).

Whilst aspects of personalisation have been welcomed both by service-user groups and professionals, its critics point out how it is used to reduce costs and inadvertently commodifies disabled people (Ferguson, 2007; Houston, 2010). Simpson and Price (2010) demonstrate how the implementation of *Valuing People* (DOH, 2001) and the *Personalisation Agenda* has the consequence of increasing levels of social exclusion, since the policy is implemented primarily to reduce costs. This becomes increasingly important within the broader welfare debate, given the declared intention of the UK's Conservative–Liberal Democrat government to reduce public expenditure by £83bn by 2014, resulting in an average 'cut' of 25% in government departments, even allowing for some protection of key areas (Elliot and Mulholland, 2010), with people with learning disabilities being targeted disproportionately (Gentleman, 2011). The impact of economic constraints in policy implementation for people with a learning disability is also not confined to England. Analysing the Polish context, where major changes had occurred following the end of Communist rule, Otrebski *et al.* (2003) show how economic factors have inhibited policy implementation most notably in relation to 'quality of life'.

Wellbeing and the Role of Social Work Education

Social work education in England is regulated by the General Social Care Council (GSCC). Through a number of specified requirements, all awards have to be subject to GSCC approval and Higher Education Institute validation. Orme and Preston-Shoot (2008), in the benchmarking standards for the BA (Social Work), refer to the different welfare traditions within the four countries of the UK, which have shaped social work education and practice. The standards do not make specific reference to named theoretical positions but identify the 'social processes associated with … disablement' (2008, p. 7) and the use of sociological, psychological and physiological perspectives (p. 9). There is also reference to the ethical principles which underpin social work practice. Whilst the references are oblique, there is sufficient there to develop the key policy areas and the dominant paradigms associated with learning disability. Finally, within social work's National Occupational Standards, people with 'learning *difficulties*' are identified as one of the 'main groups of people using services', alongside 'child care, mental health ... older people, minority and ethnic groups, drug and alcohol use, disability and impairment' (see, for example TOPPS UK Partnership, 2002, p. 20).

The *social model* of disability forms the central part of the GSCC's post-qualifying framework for social work with adults (GSCC, 2005), and is referred to as an 'embedded value' (GSCC, 2005, p. 7). The document continues:

> The aim will be to maximise as far as possible the individual's scope for making informed judgements about, and having access to, a range of choices about independent and healthy living, staying safe and participating in and contributing to society. (GSCC, 2005, pp. 7–8)

Significantly, adults with *learning* disabilities are not explicitly referred to in the document. By contrast, the guidance for the specialist award for children, young people, their families and carers mentions (albeit only the once) children with learning *difficulties* in its requirement four:

> [Social workers should identify] ... the needs of children and young people with physical impairments and/or learning difficulties (including a knowledge and understanding of how to use the services that exist to meet those needs). (GSCC, 2005, p. 11)

'Wellbeing' is absent in all the documentation and guidance, thus, for educators, the challenge is not only incorporating the concept, but on what basis. Wellbeing is frequently located within a range of psychological or psychosocial disciplines (for example, Seligman, 2002). It is also used in the public health arena, where the aim is to create and sustain a positive working environment, often alongside policies designed to improve general health (for example, smoking cessation programmes). It is multi-disciplinary, drawing upon several academic disciplines as diverse as physiology and psychology to economics (Huppert *et al.*, 2005), something it shares with social work (Trevithick, 2005). Often, the concept appears as the antithesis to mental ill-health, and part of the difficulty with the concept for social work is its close association with 'health' and the negative connotations of 'medicalised' models of intervention, of which the social model of disability provides a critique.

Towards a Role for Wellbeing in Social Work Education and Practice

Although the concept of wellbeing is largely absent in England's policy frameworks, it is beginning to emerge in social work (Jordan, 2007; Dominelli and Hackett, 2010). A justification for its inclusion is the focus upon holistic models of practice. Ng and Chan (2005, p. 70), writing in the Chinese tradition, argue for a practice based upon 'holistic wellbeing' and argue that 'wellbeing' refers to a 'positive state and growth, rather than pathological problems'. Central to this is a whole person approach, which acknowledges vulnerability and also seeks affirmation from a strengths-based perspective. This connects with existing practice models in the Western tradition which acknowledge service-users' strengths (Graybeal, 2001), and the refocusing of practice paradigms in the 1990s (Garrett, 2003). Developing critical reflection (Fook, 2002; White *et al.*, 2006; Fook and Gardner, 2007) is a feature of contemporary practice, where the concepts of wellbeing and the whole self can have a crucial role. Finally, Stevenson (2010, p. 37), in her discussion of young adults with Down syndrome in an Australian setting, argues that the 'right to freedom and wellbeing ... [is] ... global' and should 'underpin the agency of all people (with or without a disability) in all social spheres'.

Agency is central to the English policy frameworks of *Valuing People* and *Personalisation*, yet the 'freedom' it promotes is one where an undue emphasis is placed upon the 'provision' of often costly services. This privileges 'choice', one aspect of 'wellbeing', resulting in key elements, such as community integration and social relationships, being overlooked and broader 'freedoms' being lost. Consequently, provision is increasingly driven by rational cost analyses and choice leading to the reduction of the human subject to an actor driven by 'rational choice' within the confines of the economic free-market of neo-liberalism—the so-called '*homo economicus*' (Houston, 2010). In England, the role of social workers in relation to people with learning disabilities is one of rationing increasingly scarce resources (Simpson and Price, 2010). By focusing the teaching upon wellbeing, practitioners can refocus upon the whole person, and, as will be demonstrated, develop a critical response to the resource driven nature of their role.

Introducing Wellbeing into Social Work Education

Despite the complex nature of wellbeing, it is possible to identify two particular aspects which are of immediate relevance and use to social workers—subjective wellbeing and environmental indicators of wellbeing. Subjective wellbeing refers to an individual's own sense of 'happiness' and includes relationships in their widest context, something which is often referred to as social capital (Bourdieu, 1984; Putnam, 2000), and general health, including self-reported health. Other indicators of wellbeing, for example the European Social Survey commonly used in cross-national comparison, addresses the social or environmental context of the subjective state (European Social Survey, 2010). Wellbeing then is a concept which applies to the whole person, and environmental and structural factors, reflecting social work's traditional and radical concerns with the person *and* society (Price and Simpson, 2007).

To develop wellbeing as a critical tool for current practice, a teaching programme was developed which begins with subjective wellbeing and then moves outwards to engage with wider social and environmental factors. By addressing the multi-faceted aspects of wellbeing, at the intersection of the personal and the social, 'wellbeing' can be developed into a conceptual framework which begins with the core experience of the service user, a traditional social work starting point (Mayer and Timms, 1970), more recent practice handbooks and textbooks (see, Trevithick, 2005) and which then ensures its contextualisation in social structures (Price and Simpson, 2007; Ferguson, 2008).

The teaching programme utilised the wellbeing and quality of life literature, since the distinction between 'wellbeing' and 'quality of life' is blurred. The considerable overlap led Cummins (2005, p. 335) to argue that 'subjective wellbeing' is now the 'generic descriptor' although a range of terms including 'happiness', 'subjective quality of life' and 'life satisfaction' can be found.

In his review of the quality of life measurement scales, Schalock (2004), a leading researcher in the field of quality of life for people with learning disabilities, identified a prevalence of eight core elements:

> interpersonal relations, social inclusion, personal development, physical wellbeing, self-determination, material wellbeing, emotional wellbeing, and rights. (Schalock, 2004, p. 205)

Schalock suggests a three-level categorisation, beginning with subjective measures, for example 'happiness', and then arguing that there are more measurable, objective measures, for example 'engagement in everyday life and community' and 'levels of control', before identifying structural factors which can be measured, for example employment and mortality rates. Schalock also draws attention to the changing paradigms of understanding learning disability and argues that a greater emphasis upon environmental factors and rights, as well as policy objectives and their impact, has been developed. To avoid the criticism that measurement indices may 'trivialise' the concept, it is essential to balance this with individual experiences (Schalock, 2004, p. 213). Schalock and others (see Verdugo *et al.*, 2005) focus their attention upon measurement and acknowledge that relatively little attention has been paid to the role of quality of life in policy formulation, and therefore argue that a greater understanding is needed for a more informed set of policies and practices (Schalock, 2004, p. 15).

Northway and Jenkins (2003) explore the potential use of 'quality of life' in the education of learning disability nursing, and link this to the development of person-centred practice, yet little is offered in terms of constructing a model for educators to use. Thus, for those seeking to incorporate wellbeing into social work education new models need to be developed.

From the General to the Specific: Developing a Teaching Model

The first aim of introducing wellbeing into the curriculum was to build upon traditional and radical models of social work, placing the intersection of person and society at the core of practice. Second, this could then be used as a tool for critical analysis of existing policy and practice, by equipping practitioners and students with a relevant background in wellbeing alongside an exploration of the cost-cutting practice of the personalisation agenda and Houston's (2010) '*homo economicus*'. Finally, the use of environmental factors was important to counteract the claim that wellbeing could be an attempt to focus upon individuals at the expense of structure in a crude 'happiness index' (Ferguson, 2008).

The teaching model was developed around three themes, which incorporate all of Schalock's fields and draw upon other wellbeing tools and surveys—for example, the New Economics Foundation (NEF) emphasises the importance of social wellbeing in creating supportive relationships and a sense of belonging (NEF, 2009, p. 21). The three themes were:

- relationships and friendships;
- community engagement (including education, work and health); and
- structural context (Schalock, 2004, adapted).

The themes reflect core elements in social work and are readily identifiable by current practitioners, even if 'wellbeing' or 'quality of life' do not feature prominently within the social work lexicon. An important feature of the educational aspect was to equip students and practitioners with an alternative vocabulary to reflect critically upon current and future practice. This draws on aspects of critical pedagogy (Freire, 1996) and critical reflection (Fook, 2002). Through the critical examination of policy and practice throughout the course students are better equipped to become engaged practitioners, both in reclaiming social work from a narrow agenda (Ferguson, 2008) and in developing a wider policy engagement (Simpson and Connor, 2011). Thus, practitioners and students were encouraged to examine the extent to which the following areas either featured or could potentially feature in their practice, developing 'wellbeing' as a critical tool for reflection.

The teaching was supported by two additional features: the exploration of local research 'in progress' and service-user and carer inputs. The aim was to promote the concept of wellbeing as both a viable tool for assessment and as a concept to engage in a critical analysis of current policy implementation for people with learning disabilities. In addition, current research in progress (drawing on Simpson and Price, 2009), drawing upon the experiences of people with learning disabilities, was used to contextualise the concept.

Relationships and Friendships

Friendships are vital to securing a level of personal wellbeing and these feature in all of the wellbeing or quality of life measurement scales (Schalock, 2004). In the few studies which relate to any form of disability, Murphy *et al.* (2009), utilising the concept of 'living well', identify friendships and relationships as ensuring social connectedness. *Hidden Lives* (Turning Point, 2004) reported negative attitudes towards people with learning disabilities within communities and 'integration'—the aim of current policy—appeared distant. Further, it argued that social contacts of people with learning disabilities with non-disabled people were often limited to immediate or extended family and support workers. Four years later, *Valuing People Now* (DOH, 2008, p. 9) reported that 'There is evidence that people with learning disabilities have limited opportunities to build and maintain social networks and friendships'.

Simpson and Price (2009) suggest that many people with learning disabilities find friendships and emotional support from group living, and that few create and sustain friendships outside of this context. Group living, therefore, provides social relationships, which maintain a level of social interaction. 'Village communities'—criticised because of their lack of 'integration'—also provide a setting where people with learning disabilities could make and sustain meaningful social relationships (Price and Simpson, 2007). A parent/carer of a learning disabled child commented that their son's friends were almost exclusively drawn from the group of people with learning disabilities with whom he had immediate contact and the only other social relationships were with members of his immediate and extended family, echoing the findings of *Hidden Lives* (Turning Point, 2004) and *Valuing People Now* (DOH, 2008).

Service-user accounts presented during the teaching also suggested that social relationships were limited, other than the circle of learning disabled friendships generated by group living and wider 'segregated' activities within the locality. For example, all their friends were either from the group living setting, or people with whom they had contact through other specialist activities. This underlines the findings of earlier research: people with learning disabilities generally have friendships with people who have learning disabilities and their other contacts were largely limited to family and/or family friends.

This aspect of the teaching led to critical reflections on the task of promoting independence, which, whilst a positive ideal, was not premised upon ensuring supportive relationship were nurtured and maintained. The question of friendships was not a routine element in practice, giving rise to a tension between 'independence' and 'wellbeing', which became more apparent when considering the second theme of community engagement.

Community Engagement

Community engagement is a key wellbeing indicator and a feature of policy in relation to people with a learning disability. The teaching model focuses upon questions designed to explore the meaning of community more comprehensively than *Valuing People's* utopian vision. Thereby, community can be combined with wellbeing to create a lens through which current practice can be examined. An example of this is to encourage a discussion of what 'community' means to practitioners and students, exploring concepts of 'choice' and 'independence' in relation to choosing where and with whom they live.

The policy drive is towards 'community placements', usually small supported living arrangements, with a number of staff employed to provide varying levels of support. Little sustained analysis of the *quality* of both the accommodation or levels of support exists; however, the experiences of social workers suggest that there is a range of accommodation types, from people who live in houses inherited from parents, to a more typical situation of cheap rented accommodation in poorer neighbourhoods. The objective of such a policy is integration and inclusion, though as Simpson and Price (2010) demonstrate this is frequently not achieved.

Turning Point (2004) report the low levels of engagement, and consequently the high levels of isolation, experienced by many people with learning disabilities in 'community' placements. Race (2007, p. 214), a supporter of normalisation and community living, comments that 'an ordinary house is not necessarily a home'.

Choice over living location is generally not available to people with learning disabilities, due to a combination of structural factors in England: high house prices accompanied by either no or low wages for people with learning disabilities (Race, 2007, pp. 214–215).

Social isolation is significant and compounded by levels of hostility and community discrimination. Emerson *et al.* (2005) show that the utopian vision of integration into community living was far removed from the reality of daily experience for people with learning disabilities and drew attention to the importance of safety. In 2009, Fiona Pilkington, a learning disabled mother, killed herself and her disabled daughter after experiencing what was described as a 'decade of abuse' in the village in which she lived and the failure of the local council to act (Williams, 2009). This was one of the events which led to a formal inquiry by the Equality and Human Rights Commission (EHRC) into harassment and discrimination for people with disabilities. It commented that:

> Evidence already gathered by the Commission indicates that targeted violence or hostility towards disabled people is widespread in Britain. People with learning disabilities or mental health conditions in particular experience high levels of victimisation. (EHRC press release, 3 December 2009)

In September 2010, Williams reported an increase in 'mate crime'. This is a phenomenon where people with learning disabilities are targeted by others who form exploitative 'friendships' with them. Frequently the exploitation is financial, but at times results in bullying and physical or sexual violence. In the most extreme example, a man with learning disabilities who had left a small village where he grew up and was placed in a bed-sit in a larger town, was murdered by his 'mate'. The Association for Real Change (2010) has produced material to counteract the phenomenon. Through the teaching sessions it became clear that many practitioners and students were unaware of these developments and took little, if any account of them in making assessments, which were driven by 'scripted' assessment guidelines (Harris, 2003, p. 2).

The response to 'mate crime' should be in ensuring safer communities and interestingly service-user experiences from a medium sized town in the West Midlands saw good levels of integration in an area where there were significant numbers of learning disabled people. The close proximity of supported living arrangements to larger group home settings allowed groups of learning disabled people to establish a presence, which appeared to promote better community integration. Anecdotal evidence suggests that more isolated living situations were more likely to generate greater levels of intolerance (Simpson and Price, 2009). For example, one service user in 'supported living' spoke of regular harassment by the neighbours, yet by contrast, the experiences of those people living in small group homes showed good community engagement, including going to the local public house, local church groups and, perhaps most importantly, feeling safe in the local community.

In their critical reflections, practitioners and students commented that their work was dominated by the policy objective to place people within the community and that even small group homes were being targeted as 'institutions': thus, policy implementation took little account of engagement or safety, but was premised almost exclusively on location. Cree (2000) identifies location as just one aspect of defining community and adds that social networks and relationships are more important. A perceived irony is that whilst those who have real choice are frequently opting for exclusive, gated communities (for example, relatively well-off older people, and young people in modern city centre developments), similar 'communities' for people with learning disabilities are increasingly attacked for being 'segregated', yet continue to exist and have gained awards for 'sustainable communities' (Camphill Village Trust, 2010). Through a study of community and wellbeing a critical analysis develops, which allows a more fruitful exploration of both policy and practice.

Structural Context

Finally, the structural factors affecting people with learning disabilities were addressed. There are three reasons for this: first, wellbeing indicators include a range of structural factors, which enable cross-national comparisons to be undertaken, and many other factors in generating wellbeing are dependent upon this; for example, high housing costs and low income levels. By focusing upon structural factors the risks of using wellbeing as a 'happiness factor' in a non-material fashion (Ferguson, 2008) are rightly avoided. Structural factors are well documented (Turning Point, 2004; Race, 2007): whilst 40% of all people with disabilities are working, that is engaged in *some* work (The Poverty Site, 2010a), the figure for people with learning disabilities falls to under half of this at 17% (Foundation for People with Learning Disabilities, 2010), a rise from Turning Point's (2004) figure of 10%. The available data (The Poverty Site, 2010b) point to people with learning disabilities being in low-paid work or 'work experience' settings, receiving little to no remuneration. Thus, the group is largely dependent upon benefits, which are coming under attack from the UK's Conservative-led government (see earlier). The structural context is important given the now well-established argument that greater happiness and wellbeing can be found in more equal societies (Wilkinson and Pickett, 2009). The evidence provided by Race (2007) suggests that the position of people with learning disabilities is best in social democratic, more egalitarian societies.

The second 'structural factor', which needs to be considered, is a rights-based approach (see Schalock, 2004). Choice, and the ability to exercise it, is doubtless central to this and forms the premise of existing dominant paradigms (see earlier). English social work, more so than that of Scotland or Wales, is heavily influenced by promoting 'choice'. Movements towards living in the community are couched in the language of choice and empowerment—dominant and powerful concepts. There are considerable ethical considerations here, which are in danger of being reduced to the privileging of 'autonomy' as a dominant ethical value above all others. The complexities of this are beyond the scope of this paper; however, questions of choice have to be seen through the lens of wellbeing whereby a contextualisation of choice can be made to guide practice.

Third, structural factors remind practitioners and students of the two main paradigms in understanding disability discussed earlier: normalisation and the social model. Whilst the former may be more readily associated with aspects of subjective wellbeing, the limits placed upon integration were acknowledged by Nirje (1969, p. 24). He argued that normal economic standards should be applied and that work undertaken—in whatever setting—should be paid according to its worth. Oliver's materialist critique of normalisation and his promotion of the social model, drawn from Marxist sociology and its critique of capital, can be linked to structural measures of wellbeing. A focus upon wellbeing in terms of structures provides the final element in developing the 'critical tool' through education and reinforces the 'person and society' aspect of the delivery, underlining the need for a holistic approach to developing a critical and engaged practice.

Concluding Reflections

This paper has argued that 'wellbeing' provides a different and distinct lens through which social work with people with learning disabilities can be explored and has outlined how three of the prominent fields in quality of life research can be used. Through a focus upon wellbeing, practitioners and students can develop a more critical engagement with the current narrow focus of the personalisation agenda, whilst promoting the 'needs' of this service user group. Friendships, relationships and community engagement provide a challenge for social workers whose practice remains located within a narrow, resource-driven framework. This resonates with a move towards 'holistic' practice, and moreover reflects the views of the general population, where core elements of wellbeing—stability, safety, security and relationships—are highly valued. Subjective wellbeing allows social workers to focus upon individuals, and measures of national wellbeing allow them to examine social and structural factors which can have negative impacts upon people's lives. Combining subjective and structural aspects of wellbeing can create a powerful tool for critical analysis and engagement in social work education. For this to be translated into practice, further paradigm shifts in social work are needed; educating social workers prepares them to make that shift and to become part of the process of achieving it.

Note

[1] England will be the focus of analysis unless otherwise noted, since the Scottish Parliament, the Welsh Assembly and the Northern Irish power-sharing agreement have resulted in, at times subtle, at other times more substantial, differences in provision and political direction. Where 'UK' is used this is to reflect policies which are, or were, binding upon the whole Union.

References

Association for Real Change (2010) *Safety Net Project—Mate Crime* [online]. Available at: http://www.arcsafety.net/index.html, accessed 25 September 2010.

Bigby, C. & Atkinson, D. (2010) 'Written out of history: invisible women in intellectual disability social work', *Australian Social Work*, vol. 63, no. 1, pp. 4–17.

Bourdieu, P. (1984) *Distinction: A Social Critique of the Judgement of Taste*, Routledge and Kegan Paul, London.

Burton, M. & Kagan, C. (2006) 'Decoding *Valuing People*', *Disability and Society*, vol. 21, pp. 229–313.

Camphill Village Trust (2010) [online]. Available at: http://www.cvt.org.uk/botton, accessed 29 September 2010.

Cree, V. E. (2000) *Sociology for Social Workers and Probation Ofiicers*, Routledge, London.

Cummins, R. A. (2005) 'Caregivers as managers of subjective wellbeing: a homeostatic perspective', *Journal of Applied Research in Intellectual Disabilities*, vol. 18, pp. 335–344.

Department of Health (DOH) (2001) *Valuing People*, The Stationery Office, London.

Department of Health (DOH) (2008) *Valuing People Now*, The Stationery Office, London.

Dominelli, L. & Hackett, S. (2010) 'Editorial: Enhancing wellbeing: an important issue for social work', *International Social Work*, vol. 53, no. 6, pp. 755–756.

Duffy, S. (2010) *Citizenship & Community*, Centre for Welfare Reform, Sheffield.

Elliot, L. & Mulholland, H. (2010) 'Budget 2010: VAT to rise to 20% as Osborne seeks to balance books by 2015', *The Guardian*, 22 June [online]. Available at: http://www.guardian.co.uk/uk/ 2010/jun/22/budget-2010-vat-rise-osborne, accessed 30 September 2010.

Emerson, E., Malam, S., Davis, I. & Spencer, K. (2005) *Adults with Learning Difficulties in England 2003/2004 Reports*, National Statistics and NHS Health & Social Care Information Centre, London.

European Social Survey (2010) [online]. Available at: http://ess.nsd.uib.no/ess/, accessed 30 September 2010.

Ferguson, I. (2007) 'Increasing user choice or privatizing risk? The antinomies of personalization', *British Journal of Social Work*, vol. 37, pp. 387–403.

Ferguson, I. (2008) *Reclaiming Social Work*, Sage, London.

Flynn, R. J. & Lemay, R. A. (1999) *A Quarter Century of Normalization and Social Role Valorization: Evolution and Impact*, University of Ottawa Press, Ottawa.

Fook, J. (2002) *Social Work: Critical Theory and Practice*, Sage Publications, London.

Fook, J. & Gardner, F. (2007) *Critical Reflection: A Resource Handbook*, Open University Press, Maidenhead.

Foucault, M. (1979) *Discipline and Punish: The Birth of the Prison*, Vintage Books, Random House, New York.

Foundation for People with Learning Disabilities (2010) *Employment for People with Learning Disabilities* [online]. Available at: http://www.learningdisabilities.org.uk/information/issues/ education-and-employment/employment/, accessed 30 September 2010.

Freire, P. (1996) *Pedagogy of the Oppressed*, Penguin Books, London.

Garrett, P.-M. (2003) 'Swimming with dolphins: the assessment framework, New Labour and new tools for social work with children and families', *British Journal of Social Work*, vol. 33, pp. 441–463.

General Social Care Council (GSCC) (2005) *Specialist Standards and Requirements for Post-Qualifying Social Work Education and Training: Social Work with Adults*, GSCC, London.

Gentleman, A. (2011) 'Disability living allowance cuts could confine disabled to homes, say charities', *Society Guardian*, 12 January.

Graybeal, C. (2001) 'Strengths-based social work assessment: transforming the dominant paradigm', *Families in Society*, vol. 82, no. 3, pp. 233–242.

Harris, J. (2003) *The Social Work Business*, Routledge, London.

Houston, S. (2010) 'Beyond homo economicus: recognition, self-realization and social work', *British Journal of Social Work*, vol. 40, pp. 841–857.

Hreinsdottir, E. E., Stefansdottir, G., Lewthwaite, A., Ledger, S. & Shufflebotham, L. (2006) 'Is my story so different from yours? Comparing life stories, experiences of institutionalization and self-advocacy in England and Iceland', *British Journal of Learning Disability*, vol. 34, pp. 157–166.

Huppert, F. A., Bayliss, N. & Keverne, B. (eds) (2005) *The Science of Well-being*, Oxford University Press, Oxford.

Jordan, B. (2007) *Social Work and Wellbeing*, Russel House Press, Lyme Regis.

Knust-Potter, E. (1998) *Behinderung—Enthinderung. Die Community Living Bewegung gegen Ausgrenzung und Fremdbestimmung*, KNI Paperbacks, Köln.

Mayer, J. E. & Timms, N. (1970) *The Client Speaks: Working Class Impressions of Casework*, Routledge and Kegan Paul, London.

Murphy, K., Cooney, A., Shea, E. O. & Casey, D. (2009) 'Determinants of quality of life for older people living with a disability in the community', *Journal of Advanced Nursing*, vol. 65, no. 3, pp. 606–615.

New Economic Foundation (NEF) (2009) *National Accounts of Wellbeing: Bringing Real Wealth on to the Balance Sheet*, NEF, London.

Ng, S. M. & Chan, C. L. W. (2005) 'Social work intervention to embrace holistic wellbeing', in *Social Work Futures: Crossing Boundaries, Transforming Practice*, eds R. Adams, L. Dominelli & M. Payne, Palgrave Macmillan, Basingstoke, pp. 68–82.

Nirje, B. (1969) *The Normalization Principle and Its Human Management Implications*, reprinted in *The International Social Role Valorization Journal*, vol. 1, no. 1994 [online]. Available at: http://www.socialrolevalorization.com/articles/journal/1994/english/normalization-principles.pdf, accessed 24 September 2010.

Northway, R. & Jenkins, R. (2003) 'Quality of life as a concept for developing learning disability nursing practice?', *Journal of Clinical Nursing*, vol. 12, pp. 57–66.

Oliver, M. (1990) *The Politics of Disablement*, Macmillan, Basingstoke.

Oliver, M. (2001) *Capitalism, Disability and Ideology: A Materialist Critique of the Normalization Principle* [online]. Available at: http://www.leeds.ac.uk/disability-studies/archiveuk/Oliver/cap%20dis%20ideol.pdf, accessed 29 September 2010.

Orme, J. & Preston-Shoot, M. (2008) *Subject Benchmarks Statement—Social Work* [online]. Available at: http://www.qaa.ac.uk/academicinfrastructure/benchmark/statements/socialwork08.asp, accessed 30 September 2010.

Otrebski, W., Northway, R. & Mansell, I. (2003) 'Social policy and people with intellectual disabilities in Poland. Enhancing quality of life?', *Journal of Intellectual Disabilities*, vol. 7, pp. 363–374.

Price, V. & Simpson, G. (2007) *Transforming Society? Social Work and Sociology*, The Policy Press, Bristol.

Putnam, R. (2000) *Bowling Alone: The Collapse and Revival of American Community*, Simon and Schuster, New York.

Race, D. (2003) *Leadership and Change in Human Services. Selected Readings from Wolf Wolfensberger*, Routledge, London.

Race, D. (2007) *Intellectual Disability: Social Approaches*, McGraw-Hill Open University Press, Maidenhead.

Race, D., Boxall, K. & Carson, I. (2005) 'Towards a dialogue for practice: reconciling social role valorization and the social model of disability', *Disability & Society*, vol. 20, no. 5, pp. 507–521.

Rolph, S., Atkinson, D., Nind, M. & Welshman, J. (2005) *Witnesses to Change: Families, History and Learning Disability*, British Institute of Learning Disabilities, London.

Rolph, S., Atkinson, D. & Walmsey, J. (2003) 'A pair of stout shoes and an umbrella: the role of the mental welfare officer in delivering community care in East Anglia: 1946–1970', *British Journal of Social Work*, vol. 33, pp. 339–359.

Ryan, J. with Thomas, F. (1987) *The Politics of Mental Handicap*, Free Association Books, London.

Schalock, R. A. (2004) 'The concept of quality of life: what we know and do not know. Keynote address', *Journal of Intellectual Disability Research*, vol. 48, no. 3, pp. 203–216.

Seligman, M. E. P. (2002) *Authentic Happiness*, Free Press, New York.

Shakespeare, T. (2006) *Disability Rights and Wrongs*, Routledge, London.

Simpson, G. & Connor, C. (2011) *Social Policy for Welfare Professionals: Tools for Understanding, Analysis and Engagement*, The Policy Press, Bristol.

Simpson, G. & Price, V. (2009) 'Inclusive principles for social work with learning disabled people in the UK', *EASSW and ENSACT Conference* Dubrovnik, 27 April.

Simpson, G. & Price, V. (2010) 'From inclusion to exclusion: some unintended consequences of "Valuing People"', *British Journal of Learning Disabilities*, vol. 38, no. 3, pp. 180–187.

Stevenson, M. (2010) 'Flexible and responsive research: developing rights based emancipatory disability research methodology in collaboration with young adults with Down syndrome', *Australian Social Work*, vol. 63, no. 1, pp. 35–50.

The Poverty Site (2010a) *What the Indicators Show: Disability* [online]. Available at: http://www.poverty.org.uk/summary/disability.htm, accessed 9 September 2010.

The Poverty Site (2010b) *Low Income and Disability* [online]. Available at: http://www.poverty.org.uk/40/index.shtml?4, accessed 9 September 2010.

TOPPS UK Partnership (2002) *National Occupational Standards for Social Work*, TOPPS England, Leeds.

Trevithick, P. (2005) *Social Work Skills: A Practice Handbook*, Open University Press, Maidenhead.

Turning Point (2004) *Hidden Lives*, Turning Point, London.

Verdugo, M. A., Schalock, R. L., Keith, K. D. & Stancliffe, R. J. (2005) 'Quality of life and its measurement: important principles and guidelines', *Journal of Intellectual Disability Research*, vol. 49, no. 10, pp. 707–717.

White, S., Fook, J. & Gardner, F. (2006) *Critical Reflection in Health and Social Care*, Open University Press, Maidenhead.

Wilkinson, R. & Pickett, K. (2009) *The Spirit Level: Why More Equal Societies Almost Always Do Better*, Penguin Books, London.

Williams, R. (2009) 'Pilkington case may be a Lawrence moment for disability hate crime', *Society Guardian*, 28 September [online]. Available at: http://www.guardian.co.uk/uk/2009/sep/28/fiona-pilkington-inquest-disability-hate, accessed 16 September 2010.

Williams, R. (2010) '"Mate crime" fears for people with learning disabilities', *Society Guardian*, 14 September [online]. Available at: http://www.guardian.co.uk/society/2010/sep/14/learning-disabilities-mate-crime, accessed 16 September 2010.

Wolfensberger, W. (1972) *The Principle of Normalization in Human Services*, National Institute on Mental Retardation, Toronto.

World Health Organisation (WHO) (1986) *Ottawa Charter for Health Promotion* First International Conference on Health Promotion, Ottawa, 21 November, WHO/HPR/HEP/95.1.

From Theory Toward Empathic Self-Care: Creating a Mindful Classroom for Social Work Students

Maria Napoli & Robin Bonifas

Social work students experience stress, emotional exhaustion and vicarious trauma during their education; these reactions can negatively impact their ability to objectively practice and integrate course material. When social work students are mindful in the classroom, meaning they are present without internal or external filters, they are better able to regulate emotions and are more open to diverse perspectives. Teaching social work students to become mindful can improve self-care and is also the first step toward developing empathy. As such, mindful practice can help enhance practice skills, especially those related to tuning in to clients. This paper describes the elements of a mindful classroom, introduces a framework for teaching mindful practice, and presents the results of a research study that examined learning outcomes associated with this framework. Graduate students participated in a 16-week course that focused on enhancing self-care and professional development via the use of formal and informal mindful practice strategies. The Kentucky Inventory of Mindfulness Scale was administered before and after the course to assess changes in students' use of mindfulness skills. Four skill areas were tested: acting with awareness, observing, accepting without judgment, and describing; results indicate that students significantly increased their use of mindfulness in the first three areas.

Introduction

Training social workers is a challenge because the combination of science and art that characterizes professional practice is not easily taught in a classroom. Social workers provide the majority of services and referrals in health, mental health and psychology in the United States (Grant *et al.*, 2009) and most public social service administrators in the United Kingdom begin their careers as direct mental health practitioners (Pottage and Huxley, 1996). Given these realities, it is important that schools of social work provide an avenue for educating social work students in integrative health. Compared to the traditional biomedical model of disease, the integrative health model places greater emphasis on care of the whole person within a social, environmental and cultural context (Boon *et al.*, 2004). Integrative health practices stress health promotion and well-being and view the client and practitioner as partners in the healing process. Guided by the belief that people are responsible for and can positively influence their own health (Epstein, 2003a), these practices align with client empowerment, a core tenet of social work practice.

The integrative health model also recognizes the importance of practitioner self-care and asserts that neither social work students nor seasoned social workers can provide adequate services when they are tired, angry or overwhelmed (Pottage and Huxley, 1996). Teaching students the tools for mindful practice, a component of integrative health, can enable students to enhance their own self-care strategies while also improving their social work skills. Defined as the process of bringing awareness and attention to the present experience without internal or external filters (Napoli, 2010a), mindful practice is linked to a variety of positive outcomes. For example, mindfulness training among allied health students is associated with reduced stress (Rosenzweig *et al.*, 2003; Shapiro *et al.*, 2007; Carmody and Baer, 2008); reduced burnout (Moore and Cooper, 1996; Cohen-Katz *et al.*, 2005); and reduced vicarious trauma (Cunningham, 2003, 2004). In addition, it is associated with increased empathy (Beddoe and Murphy, 2004) and greater objectivity and overall quality of life (Connelly, 1999). For social work students specifically, a mindfulness-informed intervention aimed at stress reduction has been linked to significant declines in students' stress levels post training (Dziegielewski *et al.*, 2004).

This paper reviews the benefits of a mindful social work classroom, introduces a framework for teaching mindful practice to social work graduate students, and presents the results of a research study that examined learning outcomes associated with this framework. Before discussing the mindful classroom, associated course content and its subsequent impact on student learning, the role of mindfulness in developing key social work skills is detailed. Associated advantages include maximizing students' ability to begin where the client is, facilitating their recognition of countertransference reactions, minimizing the negative effects of vicarious trauma and supporting their capacity for increased empathy.

Benefits of Mindfulness in Learning Social Work Practice Skills

In mastering social work skills, the increased awareness and attention characteristic of mindful practice can help students deeply understand clients' experiences and thus more effectively begin where the client is. When students are mindful, they are aware and accepting of whatever is arising in the present moment without judgment, which strengthens their ability to understand clients' perspectives and fosters the development of a therapeutic relationship. Furthermore, mindfulness promotes self-acceptance (Carson and Langer, 2006), which can foster novice social workers' abilities to maintain focus on the client's communication and help ward off distractions associated with their own performance anxiety. Similarly, because mindful practitioners attend to their own physical and mental processes in a nonjudgmental way and use the insights gained to 'act with clarity and insight' (Epstein, 1999, p. 282), teaching social work students to mindfully monitor their personal reactions can facilitate identification of potential countertransference issues that arise during client interaction. Indeed, the self-awareness characteristic of mindful practice can enable them to recognize 'afflictive emotions before they interfere with the client–worker relationships' (Kessen, 2009, p. 42).

Research evidence describes the hazards practicing social workers face when treating traumatized clients. For example, empathetic interaction centered on another's horrific experience places practitioners at risk for increased stress, anxiety and sleep disturbances (Cunningham, 2004), as well as decreased general health (Collins and Long, 2003), emotional exhaustion and depersonalization (Moore and Cooper, 1996). Social work students also experience such vicarious trauma when introduced to distressful cases in the classroom. In fact, studies indicate that they frequently experience more emotional stress during their social work training than during their subsequent professional careers (Kramer, 1987; Tobin and Carson, 1994). They are often overwhelmed by case material, class discussions and presentations regarding clients' painful experiences, which evoke feelings and reactions that can be unfamiliar and disturbing (Cunningham, 2004). For example, after hearing a case presentation on severe child abuse, a student stated that he was unable 'to get the details out of his mind all week' (Cunningham, 2004, p. 306). Exposure to the complex problems faced by their field internship clients tends to magnify these stressful feelings (Pottage and Huxley, 1996). As such, social work students may be inundated with circumstances that elicit feelings and thoughts that may hinder their ability to be successful and that can perpetuate 'burn out' before they even graduate (Pottage and Huxley, 1996).

Research on trauma work notes the importance of educators taking steps to minimize the deleterious effects of trauma on students (Collins and Long, 2003); findings suggest the need to introduce self-care tools early in students' educational careers (Schure et al., 2008). Social work instructors can help students deal with the impact of vicarious trauma by incorporating mindful practice methods into self-care curricula; such methods can help counteract distressing experiences and thereby prevent negative outcomes. It has been suggested that quality care can only be provided when the person giving care is also well (Moore and Cooper, 1996, p. 82). We must first be mindful for ourselves before we can employ mindfulness in support of others (Williamson, 2003, p. 19). As Siegel (2010) states so eloquently, 'If we don't care for ourselves, we'll become limited in how we can care for others' (p. 3).

Evidence also suggests that when social work students are taught to mindfully reflect upon their experiences without judgment, their capacity for empathy can increase. For example, a study of nursing students trained in mindfulness found a decrease in personal distress and an increase in qualities associated with fostering empathy (Beddoe and Murphy, 2004). Indeed, mindful reflection intensifies the activity in the prefrontal cortex and 'this neural integration promotes a reflective mind, an adaptive, resilient brain and empathic relationships' (Siegel, 2007, p. 262). In addition, when social work students and educators are mindfully in tune with each other, students' ability for authenticity in classroom interactions can increase, creating additional opportunities for greater empathy.

Through mindful practice, social work students can intentionally pay attention without judgment to what is happening with them, both in the classroom and in client interactions. This offers them opportunities to become resilient and, within a safe environment, to confront the challenges they will face in practice. By creating a mindful classroom, students may be better able to increase overall self-care by making constructive changes in their personal and professional lives. The components of a mindful classroom are reviewed below.

Elements of the Mindful Classroom

The mindful classroom takes students out of the book and into self-reflection by stimulating their creativity and passion, opening the door for active and engaged learning. Social work educators can create stimulating learning environments by emphasizing the following elements of the mindful classroom: empathically acknowledging; intentionally paying attention; accepting experience without judgment; and enhancing sensory awareness. These elements work together to enable students to develop objectivity and resiliency toward adjusting to change.

Empathically acknowledging one's experience, often by putting it into words, is the first step toward mindfulness. Students need permission to acknowledge their thoughts, emotions and biases not only toward themselves, but also toward the clients they serve. This sets the stage for honesty and clarity in approaching one's experience, which reduces the likelihood of offering clients non-genuine responses. Indeed, it has been found that mindful students are more authentic in their interactions with others (Carson and Langer, 2006); such authenticity is an important criterion in building trusting relationships with clients. To support students' ability to acknowledge their experience, social work educators must first create a safe environment for students to express their fears and doubts verbally or in writing while seeking solutions to problems. A protected setting enables students to develop competence by helping them to gain knowledge and strengthen their capacity to adapt to change (Epstein, 2003b).

Intentionally paying attention to one's experience gives students a plethora of information on how they are either reacting or responding to their experiences. Noticing such things as breath, body, emotions and thoughts may take a few more moments before acting upon information given, yet the self-awareness achieved is invaluable to enhancing the quality of interactions with clients. When students intentionally pay attention to what they are experiencing in the present moment, they are better able to listen before expressing an opinion, and thereby bring a more heartfelt nature into their communications. While technique and theory are vital components of effective social work practice, when students are taught to focus on curricula and behavior in lieu of consciousness, they close their minds to equally important ideas and feelings (Epstein, 1999). If students are not paying attention to how they are reacting, it not only fosters perpetuation of those emotions, but also stagnates imagination and curiosity, which are key components for integration and transfer of knowledge learned. Understanding and having insights about oneself are not enough for social work students to practice; they need to be able to incorporate what they have learned into daily living and explore the meaning of their emotions that arise.

Mindful students are better able to *accept their experience without judgment* and, as noted above, can increase their propensity for empathy by doing so. Empathy turned toward oneself enables one to revisit or experience an event or affect without judgment (Morgan and Morgan, 2005, p. 83); when students can accept themselves without judgment, their capacity to accept others increases. Indeed, neuroscientists describe a phenomenon whereby neurons involved in various daily activities are stimulated in our own brains when we simply observe another individual engaged in that activity (Siegel, 2007). This 'mirror neuron' system is directly involved in feeling empathy; by practicing mindfulness we can actually stimulate these mirror neurons (Siegel, 2007).

As such, an important route to developing empathy is *sensory awareness*. Mindfully using all of our senses helps gain information about our experience and deepens our awareness of what is happening in that experience. In addition, non-verbal messages represent the first and the most internalized information we receive when interacting with another, thus sensation is intimately connected with the brain's empathy pathways. Mindfulness increases our attention to sensations, which helps engage those mirror neurons. When students are mindful and pay attention to their senses and associated instincts, increased empathy can ensue.

As social work students develop their mindful practice by empathically acknowledging, intentionally paying attention, accepting their experience without judgment and enhancing sensory awareness, the window of opportunity for taking action toward change increases. Teaching social work students mindfulness helps them view a client's problem from a new perspective because thoughts and emotions are perceived without judgment and thus, are not censored. There is a difference between teaching students to be competent versus teaching them to be capable. Competence can be viewed as what people know or what they are able to do, but capability is the extent to which individuals can adapt to change, generate new knowledge and continue to improve their performance (Epstein, 2003b, p. 11). Mindfulness offers students this capability to be resilient and open to change, which creates maximum opportunity for learning. When students mindfully move away from scripted responses in the classroom they are better able to offer a more genuine response and consider various solutions to the situation (Carson and Langer, 2006). It is essential that instructors develop a classroom that allows for critical and creative thinking so students can move from rigid personal and theoretical ideas to openness of new ideas where learning is self-directed. One method for striving to accomplish this, a course entitled *Quality of Life,* is detailed below.

Creating a Mindful Classroom: The *Quality of Life* Curriculum

Quality of Life is a 16-week graduate course that facilitates students' personal exploration of self-care and enables them to witness their own experience such that they respond to situations instead of reacting to them. A primary goal of the course is to support students in gaining mindfulness practice skills, such that they can make changes in self-care strategies that improve their overall health and well-being. The *Quality of Life* course emphasizes the four elements of mindfulness described above and guides students in employing these elements to take action toward change by fostering openness to new ideas. Teaching students how to respond rather than react to the core issues in their lives increases the possibility of empathy, clarity and harmony.

Essential Skill Taught: Breath Awareness

Conscious awareness of the breath is a fundamental mindfulness skill that helps students focus; therefore, breathing activities are incorporated throughout each class session. Beginning the class with a 10-minute mindful breathing meditation enables students to quiet their busy minds and pay attention to the task at hand in the 'here and now'. In addition, later on in the class session when considerable information is being presented and overlapping dialogue occurs, students again engage in a brief one- to two-minute mindful breathing exercise. This silent reflection can reduce students' confusion and frustration and give them a quiet moment to reconnect since consciously paying attention to the breath facilitates focusing and a sense of calm alertness. Furthermore, it creates the opportunity for deeper understanding and more coherent expression of thoughts (Zinger, 2008, p. 26). Students are also reminded throughout the semester to bring attention to the breath in their daily routines at home, school and at field internship or work.

Class Format and Learning Activities

Class meets weekly for a three-hour block. Each week students participate in classroom activities that focus on a different aspect of self-care. Example topics include nutrition, exercise, creating healthy relationships and environments, exploring passions and intentionally exploring vision. In conjunction with each self-care topic, students read journal articles related to the topic and complete critical thinking logs that reflect their thoughts and opinions of the material as well as how each topic relates to their lives. Students also complete a weekly journal describing their use of mindful practice at home, school, and field internship or work. They are given freedom to express how their mindfulness practice impacted on them through art, poetry, ideas and feelings, as well as simple narrative descriptions of their mindful practice experience.

Outside of the classroom, students engage in a one-hour mindfulness practice twice a week using an audio mindfulness practice tool: *Tools for Mindful Living: Stepping Stones for Practice CD* (Napoli, 2010b). The CD walks students through the process of various mindful practice activities. Students also complete mindfulness exercises in two workbooks, *Tools for Mindful Living: Steppingstones for Practice* (Napoli, 2010a) and *Life by Personal Design: Choices or Consequences* (Napoli and Roe, 2008). These exercises focus on skill development in terms of quality of life, self-care and mindfulness practice; detailed examples of the exercises are available from the first author.

At the end of the semester, students participate in a closing ritual: a mindfulness silent meal, where each student contributes food in a buffet style, creating a sensory experience of viewing the table spread with food, touching, smelling, hearing sounds while chewing and, of course, tasting the food. This is followed by a discussion of the sensory experience.

The next section details learning outcomes associated with students' participation in the *Quality of Life* course.

Method

Two research questions informed the evaluation of the *Quality of Life* curriculum: (1) after completing the course, do students report more frequent use of mindful practice strategies compared to their baseline usage before exposure to the *Quality of Life* curriculum?; and (2) after completing the course, do students report using some mindfulness practices more often than others compared to their usage before exposure to the *Quality of Life* curriculum? A cross-sectional pre-test/post-test research design was utilized to gain insight into the answers to these questions.

Data Collection

Data were collected in two course sections of *Quality of Life*. The Kentucky Inventory of Mindfulness questionnaire (Baer *et al.*, 2004), described below, was administered to students at three time points: the beginning of the course (pre-test), the end of the course (post-test), and six months following the completion of the course (follow-up). Response rates at the six-month follow-up were insufficient such that associated data are not included in this analysis; this suggests an additional incentive is needed to prompt students to return questionnaires after completing the course.

Measures

The Kentucky Inventory of Mindfulness (KIMS) scale was utilized to capture students' mastery of mindful practice strategies. The KIMS was developed to measure the use of mindful practices in daily life among both general and clinical populations (Baer *et al.*, 2004). The questionnaire contains 39 items measured on a five-point scale where 1 = Never or rarely true, 2 = Rarely true, 3 = Sometimes true, 4 = Often true, and 5 = Very often or always true. Example items include 'I notice how food and drinks affect my thoughts, bodily sensations, and emotions' and 'I notice changes in my body such as whether my breathing slows down or speeds up'. A description of each KIMS item is available in Baer *et al.*, (2004).

The scale developers conceptualized mindfulness as a multidimensional construct; exploratory and confirmatory factor analysis revealed the presence of four mindfulness dimensions: observing (12 items); describing (eight items), acting with awareness (10 items), and accepting without judgment (nine items). Cronbach's alphas for each scale in the study sample were 0.91, 0.84, 0.83, and 0.87, respectively. *Observing* captures the ability to pay attention to internal and external stimuli, such as cognitions and sounds, as in the example question 'I pay attention to whether my muscles are tense or relaxed'. *Describing* captures the tendency to put experiences and thoughts into words, as in the example question 'I'm good at finding the words to describe my feelings'. *Acting with awareness* taps the ability to focus attention on a current activity, for example 'When I do things, my mind wanders off and I'm easily distracted'. *Accepting without judgment* measures tendencies to criticize one's thoughts, emotions, and experiences; for example 'I tell myself that I shouldn't be thinking what I'm thinking'. While other mindfulness measures exist, the KIMS was selected because these subscales directly correspond to the elements of the mindful classroom described above: empathically acknowledging (i.e. *Describing*), intentionally paying attention (i.e. *Acting with awareness*), accepting experience without judgment (i.e. *Accepting without judgment*), and enhancing sensory awareness (i.e. *Observing*).

The KIMS was normed using a sample of diverse undergraduate psychology students ($n = 420$) and a clinical sample of individuals diagnosed with borderline personality disorder ($n = 26$); psychometric testing revealed strong content validity, high internal consistency, and adequate test–retest reliability (Baer *et al.*, 2004).

Data Analysis

Predictive Analytics Software Statistics (PASW, formally SPSS) version 18 was utilized for all statistical calculations. Data were first screened for errors, outliers, and missing data. Of the 48 students, 46 provided data on the KIMS during class sessions, representing a 95.8% response rate; however, 15 questionnaires were largely incomplete. These cases are not included in the analysis, resulting in a final sample size of 31. The majority of variables had one or two cases with missing data, contributing to 7.14% missing data overall; missing data were imputed using a linear interpolation method to allow scale construction for all respondents in the sample. Consistent with the KIMS, 18 questionnaire items were reverse coded to facilitate interpretation of results and comparison across items.

Results

Sample

Since the primary focus of data collection was assessing the impact of the course content overall, student demographics were not collected via the individual surveys.

However, to provide a context for understanding the population of students enrolled in *Quality of Life*, 85.4% were female ($f = 41$) and 85.4% were Caucasian. Four students were Latino, one was Native American, and two were African American.

Research Question 1: Changes in Use of Mindfulness Strategies Before and After Exposure to Quality of Life Curriculum

To determine whether or not students' responses to the KIMS changed in association with exposure to the *Quality of Life* curriculum, the 39 items on the KIMS were first reduced into the four subscales identified by Baer *et al.*, (2004). At pre-test, students scored highest on the *Accepting without judgment* scale ($M = 3.46$; $SD = 0.68$), followed by the *Observing* scale ($M = 3.38$; $SD = 0.72$) and the *Describing* scale ($M = 3.37$; $SD = 0.89$). Students scored the lowest on the *Acting with awareness* scale ($M = 2.87$; $SD = 0.61$).

Paired-sample *t*-tests were then calculated for each of the four subscales (Table 1). Results indicated that students made statistically significant gains in three of the mindfulness domains: *Accepting without judgment* ($p < 0.05$), *Acting with awareness* ($p < 0.001$), and *Observing* ($p < 0.001$). Statistically significant gains were not made on the *Describing* domain.

Research Question 2: Are Some Mindfulness Practice Strategies Used More Often Than Others After Exposure to Quality of Life *Curriculum?*

Mean scores were calculated for all KIMS items to assess students' areas of strength and weakness in mindful practice at pre-test (Table 2). To minimize errors associated with multiple *t*-tests and for brevity, interest focused on the five highest and lowest extremes. Given the coding scheme noted above, with lower numbers corresponding to lower mindfulness attributes and higher numbers corresponding to higher mindfulness attributes, positive values represent improvement in mindfulness practice (Table 2).

Results indicate that students made the largest gains on four single items from the *Observing* scale and one from the *Describing* scale: 'I pay attention to whether my muscles are tense or relaxed' (mean diff = 1.16; $SD = 1.13$); 'I notice how foods and drinks affect my thoughts, bodily sensations, and emotions' (mean diff = 1.13;

Table 1 Differences in Mean Mindfulness Subscale Scores over Time ($n = 31$)

Domain	Pre-test	SD	Post-test	SD	t
Accepting without judgment	3.46	0.68	3.71	0.74	2.127*
Acting with awareness	2.87	0.61	3.29	0.40	4.944***
Describing	3.37	0.89	3.49	0.54	0.678
Observing	3.38	0.72	4.25	0.56	6.103***

Notes: *$p < 0.05$, **$p < 0.01$, ***$p < 0.001$.

Table 2 Areas of Greatest and Least Change on Individual Mindfulness Items ($n = 31$)

Item	Mean time 1	SD	Mean time 2	SD	Mean difference	t
Greatest Improvement						
Attention to muscle tension (Observing)	3.23	1.02	4.39	0.67	1.16	5.730***
Notice affect of foods and drinks (Observing)	2.94	1.09	4.06	0.73	1.13	5.479***
Awareness of feelings (Observing)	3.13	1.06	4.19	0.70	1.06	22.25***
Notice bodily changes (Observing)	3.23	1.02	4.26	0.88	1.03	5.657***
Tendency to put experiences into words (Describing)	3.13	1.12	4.10	1.14	0.97	4.991***
Least Improvement						
Difficulty describing sensations (Describing)[a]	3.48	1.12	3.65	1.20	0.16	0.681
Belief that some thoughts are bad (Accepting without judgment)[a]	3.94	0.81	4.10	0.83	0.16	0.961
Trouble finding words to express feelings (Describing)[a]	3.68	1.08	3.84	1.10	0.16	0.961
Tendency to evaluate perceptions. (Accepting without judgment)[a]	2.61	1.05	2.74	0.96	0.13	0.680
Notice mood changes (Observing)	3.97	0.79	4.06	0.85	0.09	0.571

Notes: *$p < 0.05$, **$p < 0.01$, ***$p < 0.001$
[a]Reverse-coded item.

$SD = 1.15$); 'I intentionally stay aware of my feelings' (mean diff $= 1.06$; $SD = 0.96$); 'I notice changes in my body such as whether my breathing slows down or speeds up' (mean diff $= 1.03$; $SD = 1.02$); and 'My natural tendency is to put my experiences into words' (mean diff $= 0.97$; $SD = 1.08$).

Minimal gains were made in two individual items on the *Accepting without judgment* scale, one on the *Observing* scale, and two on the *Describing* scale, specifically: 'When I have a sensation in my body, it's difficult for me to describe it because I can't find the right words' (mean diff $= 0.16$; $SD = 1.32$); 'I believe some of my thoughts are abnormal or bad and I shouldn't think that way' (mean diff $= 0.16$; $SD = 0.93$); 'I have trouble thinking of the right words to express how I feel about things' (mean diff $= 0.16$; $SD = 0.93$); 'I tend to evaluate whether my perceptions are right or wrong' (mean diff $= 0.13$; $SD = 1.06$); and 'I notice when my mood begins to change' (mean diff $= 0.09$; $SD = 0.94$).

Discussion

These findings indicate that participation in the *Quality of Life* course is associated with statistically significant improvement in three of the four components of mindfulness: *Observing*, *Acting with awareness*, and *Accepting without judgment*; it is not associated with statistically significant gains in *Describing*. Prior to exposure to the mindfulness curriculum, students tended to score higher on individual items from the *Accepting without judgment* scale and continued to develop their skills in this area as evidenced by significant improvements in the overall measure at post-test. Interestingly, students tended to score lower on several individual items of the *Acting with awareness* scale at pre-test, but were able to make considerable gains in this area at post-test. Students made the largest overall improvement in mindfulness skills related to *Observing*, with an average 0.87 gain in mean scores from pre-test to post-test. Progress in both *Acting with awareness* and *Observing* may be connected to the emphasis on attending to bodily signals in the mindfulness curriculum. However, it is important to note that a specific area in which students made minimal improvement is an item from the *Observing* scale associated with recognizing changes in their mood. This suggests that students may find paying attention to their own emotional state more difficult to master than attending to physical sensations.

Similarly, two specific areas of minimal improvement correspond to items on the *Accepting without judgment* scale and relate to students' tendency to negatively evaluate their thoughts and perceptions. Although statistically significant gains were made in the *Accepting without judgment* scale overall, students may experience more challenge in tolerating thoughts they perceive as aberrant. Students also did not make statistically significant gains on the *Describing* scale and two of the specific minimal improvement areas correspond to items on this scale. Interestingly however, one of the strongest areas of increase is in students' perception that they have a natural ability to put their experiences into words. This suggests that although students continue to struggle with the process of labeling their experiences, they perhaps feel more comfortable with the idea of doing so.

Limitations

As with all research, this study is not without limitations. Foremost, it is important to recognize that the study design is cross-sectional, thus causation cannot be ascertained and the relationships found here are correlational at best. The absence of a comparison group means the possibility cannot be ruled out that social work students naturally improve in mindfulness skills as they progress through the social work curriculum. In addition, because data were collected during class sessions in a course for which students were receiving a grade, even though questionnaires were completed anonymously, social desirability may have entered into their response patterns. In spite of these limitations, the results of this study add weight to the assertion that the *Quality of Life* curriculum can help social work students gain skills in mindful practice.

Implications

Social work students cannot develop empathy, emotional regulation and attentive listening skills by reading a book; thus, creating a mindful classroom where students can develop the skills necessary to become effective social work practitioners is important. Students in the *Quality of Life* course were able to make statistically significant gains in acting with awareness. Paying attention to body sensations, particularly one's practice instincts or 'gut feelings', is a valuable tool for social work students to possess. Indeed, Amrit Desai (2003), an enlightened spiritual leader said, 'If you listen and pay attention to your body you never have to read another book'. This ability is also one of the most difficult to acquire. During *Quality of Life*, students were guided to consciously notice sensations during formal meditation sessions as well as informally during daily life activities. Through the development of acting with awareness, students appeared to begin building upon their skills for practice in ways that may never have occurred if they remained stuck in mindlessness.

Although students were able to increase their ability to accept without judgment, they continued to struggle with verbally expressing their experiences and perceptions. Taking the awareness and being able to express that awareness helps students to control impulsivity and reactivity, thereby increasing the ability to genuinely respond to both themselves and their clients with greater empathy. Given the importance of empathetically acknowledging one's experience and describing it with words for engaging with clients authentically, findings suggest the *Quality of Life* curriculum may need additional refinement to better enable students to master this critical mindfulness skill.

In light of students' difficulty with *describing*, research indicates that although many mental health practitioners have a personal history of trauma, they are often uncomfortable talking about their traumatic experiences (Cunningham, 2004). For example, a study of psychiatrists found the stigma they felt due to depression predicted reduced help-seeking behavior (Adams *et al.*, 2010). Similarly, social work students may readily discuss how to deal with a client's problem, yet are less likely to discuss their own challenges. For instance, in a family practice class students were asked how they were feeling following a case filled with emotional content. Most of the students discussed ways to help the client as if they did not hear the question; their expectation was to 'fix' the client (Berceli and Napoli, 2006). At the same time, a course designed to teach graduate social work students the 'use of self' was ranked among the top courses taught in one MSW program (Chapman *et al.*, 2003). This apparent mismatch suggests that students want to master self-awareness skills, but need sensitive and specific guidance in doing so. Holistic reflective practitioners pay attention to the process as well as the content (Ruch, 2005, p. 117) and are thereby able to respond to and survive emotionally charged work. As such, one way that we may help social work students to express their challenges more openly is to bring them into small groups for discussions of their personal process with the clear understanding that there is *no judgment* regardless of what they think or feel. It is critical to remind students that having thoughts and feelings are very different from acting upon them.

Prior research has found that with mindful practice one tends to approach rather than withdraw from challenges. For example, mindfulness activates the left frontal area of the cerebral cortex that is related to approaching, versus the right frontal activation that is associated with withdrawal from novelty or challenges (Siegel, 2010, p. 28). Taking this into consideration, it makes sense that training social work students in mindful awareness practices is a valuable addition to their professional development. Attention to one's experience, simply noticing what you are doing now, sounds easy, yet in practice it is often a challenge with the constant distractions and interruptions inherent to everyday life. Yet students who are able to focus and pay attention to their thoughts, emotions and routines deepen their experience. Indeed, when students are mindful they are able to engage as reflective learners from a theoretical, personal, practical, critical and process perspective; seeing situations from multiple viewpoints and thinking about what they are doing while they are doing it maximizes learning (Ruch, 2000, p. 100).

As a result of our experience with students in the *Quality of Life* course, it appears that the curriculum described is a promising tool for enhancing social work students' abilities to increase their use of mindfulness skills for personal and professional use. These skills have implications for self-care, minimizing burnout, reducing stress, as well as increasing empathy, attention and objectivity in practice. Teaching students how to be mindful has the potential to not only enable them to be present for themselves and clients, but modeling mindfulness can offer clients lifelong tools to manage the change in their lives: 'The only way to comprehend mindfulness is to practice it' (Sitzman, 2002, p. 121). What better place to begin this practice than the social work classroom?

Acknowledgements

The authors would like to thank Dr Mary Gillmore for her thoughtful recommendations on developing this manuscript and Samuel Chates for his assistance in preparing the final version.

References

Adams, E. F. M., Lee, A. J., Pritchard, C. W. & White, R. J. E. (2010) 'What stops us from healing the healers: a survey of help-seeking behavior, stigmatization and depression within the medical profession', *International Journal of Social Psychiatry*, vol. 56, no. 4, pp. 359–370.

Baer, R. A., Smith, G. T. & Allen, K. B. (2004) 'Assessment of mindfulness by self report: the Kentucky Inventory of Mindfulness Skills', *Assessment*, vol. 11, no. 3, pp. 191–206.

Beddoe, A. E. & Murphy, S. O. (2004) 'Does mindfulness decrease stress and foster empathy among nursing students?', *Journal of Nursing Education*, vol. 43, no. 7, pp. 305–312.

Berceli, D. & Napoli, M. (2006) 'Mindfulness-based trauma-prevention program for social work professionals', *Journal of Complementary Health Practice Review*, vol. 11, no. 3, pp. 153–165.

Boon, H., Verhoef, M., O'Hara, D. & Findlay, B. (2004) 'From parallel practice to integrative health care: a conceptual framework', *BMC Health Services Research*, vol. 4, no. 15, doi:10.1186/1472-6963-4-15.

Carmody, J. & Baer, R. A. (2008) 'Relationships between mindfulness practice and levels of mindfulness, medical and psychological symptoms and well-being in a mindfulness-based stress reduction program', *Journal of Behavioral Medicine*, vol. 31, no. 1, pp. 22–33.

Carson, S. H. & Langer, L. (2006) 'Mindfulness and self-acceptance', *Journal of Rational-Emotive and Cognitive-Behavior Therapy*, vol. 24, no. 1, pp. 29–43.

Chapman, M. V., Oppenheim, S., Shibusawa, T. & Jackson, H. M. (2003) 'What we bring to practice: teaching students about professional use of self', *Journal of Teaching in Social Work*, vol. 23, no. 3/4, pp. 3–14.

Cohen-Katz, J., Wiley, S. D., Capuano, T., Baker, D. M. & Shapiro, S. (2005) 'The effects of mindfulness-based stress reduction on nurse stress and burnout, part 11: a quantitative and qualitative study', *Holistic Nursing Practice*, vol. 19, no. 1, pp. 26–35.

Collins, S. & Long, A. (2003) 'Too tired to care? The psychological effects of working with trauma', *Journal of Psychiatric and Mental Health Nursing*, vol. 10, no. 1, pp. 17–27.

Connelly, J. (1999) 'Being in the present moment: developing the capacity for mindfulness in medicine', *Academic Medicine*, vol. 74, no. 4, pp. 420–424.

Cunningham, M. (2003) 'Impact of trauma work on social work clinicians: empirical findings', *Social Work*, vol. 48, no. 4, pp. 451–459.

Cunningham, M. (2004) 'Teaching social workers about trauma: reducing the risks of vicarious traumatization in the classroom', *Journal of Social Work Education*, vol. 40, no. 2, pp. 305–317.

Desai, A. (2003) *Kripalu Yoga Teacher's Conference Speech*, Lenox, MA.

Dziegielewski, S. F., Roest-Marti, S. & Turnage, B. (2004) 'Addressing stress with social work students: a controlled evaluation', *Journal of Social Work Education*, vol. 40, no. 1, pp. 105–119.

Epstein, R. M. (1999) 'Mindful practice', *Journal of the American Medical Association*, vol. 282, no. 9, pp. 833–839.

Epstein, R. M. (2003a) 'Mindful practice in action (1): technical competence, evidence-based medicine, and relationship-centered care', *Families, Systems and Health*, vol. 21, no. 1, pp. 2–9.

Epstein, R. M. (2003b) 'Mindful practice in action (11): cultivation habits of mind', *Families, Systems and Health*, vol. 21, no. 1, pp. 11–17.

Grant, L., Gioia, D., Benn, R. & Seabury, B. (2009) 'Incorporating integrative health services in social work education', *Journal of Social Work Education*, vol. 45, no. 3, pp. 407–424.

Kessen, C. (2009) 'Living fully: mindfulness practices for everyday life', in *Mindfulness and Social Work*, ed. S. F. Hick, Lyceum Books, Chicago, IL.

Kramer, M. (1987) 'Comparative stress levels in part time and full time social work programs', *Journal of Social Work Education*, vol. 23, no. 3, pp. 74–80.

Moore, K. A. & Cooper, C. L. (1996) 'Stress in mental health professionals: a theoretical overview', *International Journal of Social Psychiatry*, vol. 42, no. 2, pp. 82–89.

Morgan, W. D. & Morgan, S. T. (2005) 'Cultivating attention and empathy', in *Mindfulness and Psychotherapy*, eds C. K. Germer, R. D. Siegel & R. R. Fulton, The Guildford Press, New York.

Napoli, M. (2010a) *Tools for Mindful Living: Steppingstones for Practice*, Kendall/Hunt Publishing, Dubuque, IA.

Napoli, M. (2010b) *Tools for Mindful Living: Steppingstones for Practice CD*, Kendall/Hunt Publishing, Dubuque, IA.

Napoli, M, & Roe, S. (2008) *Life by Personal Design: Choice or Consequences*, Kendall/Hunt Publishing, Dubuque, IA.

Pottage, D. & Huxley, P. (1996) 'Stress and mental health social work: a developmental perspective', *International Journal of Social Psychiatry*, vol. 42, no. 2, pp. 124–131.

Rosenzweig, S., Reibel, D. K., Greeson, J. M., Brainard, G. C. & Hojat, M. (2003) 'Mindfulness-based stress reduction lowers psychological distress in medical students', *Teaching and Learning in Medicine*, vol. 15, no. 2, pp. 88–92.

Ruch, G. (2000) 'Self and social work: towards an integrative model of learning', *Journal of Social Work Practice*, vol. 14, no. 2, pp. 99–112.

Ruch, G. (2005) 'Relationship-based practice and reflective practice: holistic approaches to contemporary child care social work', *Child and Family Social Work*, vol. 10, no. 2, pp. 111–123.

Schure, M. B., Chriostopher, J. & Christopher, S. (2008) 'Mind–body medicine and the art of self care: teaching mindfulness to counseling students through yoga, meditation and Qigong', *Journal of Counseling and Development*, vol. 86, no. 1, pp. 47–56.

Shapiro, S. L., Brown, W. K. & Biegel, G. (2007) 'Teaching self-care to caregivers: effects of mindfulness-based stress reduction on the mental health of therapist in training', *Training and Education in Professional Psychology*, vol. 1, no. 2, pp. 105–115.

Siegel, D. J. (2007) *The Mindful Brain: Reflection and Attunement in the Cultivation of Well-Being*, W.W. Norton and Co, New York.

Siegel, D. J. (2010) *The Mindful Therapist: A Clinician's Guide to Mindsight and Neural Integration*, W.W. Norton and Co, New York.

Sitzman, K. L. (2002) 'Interbeing and mindfulness: a bridge to understanding Jean Watson's theory of human caring', *Nursing Education Perspectives*, vol. 23, no. 3, pp. 118–123.

Tobin, P. J. & Carson, J. (1994) 'Stress and the student social worker', *Social Work and Social Sciences Review*, vol. 5, no. 3, pp. 246–255.

Williamson, P. R. (2003) 'Mindfulness in medicine, mindfulness in life', *Families, Systems and Health*, vol. 21, no. 1, pp. 18–20.

Zinger, L. (2008) 'Educating for tolerance and compassion: is there a place for meditation in a college classroom?', *College Teaching Methods and Styles Journal*, vol. 4, no. 4, pp. 25–28.

The Feeling of Being a Social Worker: Including Yoga as an Embodied Practice in Social Work Education

Jo Mensinga

As a social work educator and yoga teacher, I have found it curious that the body and embodied knowledge have not been the subject of more debate in the social work literature or focus in professional training. In general where and when the body is mentioned, authors either provide a note of caution warning the practitioner against relying on the body as a source of knowledge and/or a reminder that, as an object, the body has been the cause of much social oppression. Yet, much of social work practice is underpinned by the practitioner's visceral experience. For example, in the process of gathering data to complete a biopsychosocial assessment of a presenting issue that will both inform and guide any intervention strategy, the social worker must navigate both community and clients' physical spaces while negotiating their own somatic maps. Whereas social work education focuses on developing the cognitive and discursive aspects of self-awareness and reflection, recent neuroscientific studies confirm what has long been known in Eastern embodied practices, that the body is the 'main channel for influencing the mind'. Drawing on the literature exploring the mind–body connection interspersed with my own experience using yoga as a reflexive practice, I argue that making the role of the body more visible in the professional discourse and placing a greater emphasis on embodied knowledge in social work education strengthens the reflexive capacity of future practitioners leading to a greater health and well-being of social workers and better outcomes for their clients.

Introduction

> ... we have to keep in mind that the knowledge about the body is not necessarily embodied and the engagement in bodily practices or promotion of bodily practices does not alone guarantee the construction of an embodied subjectivity. On the contrary, the body is often disciplined to objectify the self under discursive

construction ... but knowing our bodies can create a more holistic self understanding. (Markula, 2004, pp. 74–75)

Despite a growing awareness of the role of embodied knowledge and the impact of neuroscience in other disciplines [e.g. psychotherapy (Rothschild, 2000), psychology (Goleman, 2006), education (Bresler, 2004) and sociology (Crossley, 2001; Howson and Inglis, 2001)], there is little exploration or research into the body–mind connection in social work theory, how it impacts practice nor how it influences the education process. When exploring the social work literature, it seems that although the body is recognised as an essential component of 'nonverbal' communication in micro skill training and/or discussed as a part of the 'use of self' when exploring the professional persona, it is rarely mentioned as a source of theorising or explored as an integral component of reflective practice (Saleebey, 1992; Peile, 1998; Tangenberg and Kemp, 2002). While Cameron and McDermott (2007, pp. 13–15) claim that there have been valid reasons for this professional disregard (e.g. that the body itself is difficult to define and much discrimination has occurred on the basis of biological characteristics), the authors also maintain that separating the mind and body veils human lived experience and ignores many of the recent neuroscientific findings that could be useful in addressing practice approaches and client inequities.

Added to emerging neuroscientific findings of how human minds are more than just our brains and that the brain/body can shape as well as be shaped by their interactions with significant others and their environments (van der Kolk, 1994; Damasio, 1999; Siegel, 2010a, 2010b), there has been growing evidence that those who work with clients who have been traumatised are more likely to develop Secondary Traumatic Stress (STS) and/or Compassion Fatigue than people in the general population (Bride and Figley, 2007; Badger et al., 2008). Not only are human service workers at risk of being physically and verbally abused, social workers are also at risk of being affected vicariously (Stanley and Goddard, 2002; Pryce et al., 2007; Koritsas et al., 2010). Interestingly, while social work students are required to develop a reflexive practice and social workers are encouraged to make use of professional supervision and/or 'talk therapies' to review their work practices, there is mounting proof that being comfortable in the body is a necessary precursor for reflection and many problem solving activities. Van der Kolk (1994) explains that memories become stored in the body and that most trauma sensitive people require some sort of body work 'to regain a sense of safety in their bodies' before they can engage in verbal reflection. While it is acknowledged that there are no actual mechanisms in the body itself that store experiences, there is evidence of an ongoing dialogue between the body and the brain that creates emotional maps that can either preserve or change specific behavioural patterns (Damasio, 1999).

Eastern embodied practices, of which yoga I am most familiar, have long claimed that the body is the 'main channel for influencing the mind' (Pagis, 2009, p. 272). Like the mindfulness practices that have become popular as psychological interventions in the last decade, yoga encourages the individual to break habitual embodied feedback loops through a process of introspection on the human body (Satterfield, 2010;

Stone, 2010). Although postural yoga has not been taken up to the same extent nor is as well researched as mindfulness in the human services sector (Shapiro and Carlson, 2009), there is increasing evidence that yoga has the potential to increase participants' awareness of their bodies, thoughts, emotions and patterns of cognition, as well as calming their central nervous system, reducing anxiety, mental stress and fatigue (Valente and Marotta, 2005). Given the accepted importance of reflection in social work practice and the current understandings emerging from the neuroscientific literature, in this article I draw attention to the emerging presence of the body in the social work literature; explore the importance of the visceral experience of the social work experience; and suggest that embodied practices such as yoga should be incorporated into academic courses to facilitate self-reflective processes in order to better prepare social work students to take care of themselves and assist improved outcomes for their clients.

Becoming Aware of the Body in the Social Work Literature

> While you read this paragraph take note of what bodily sensations you are experiencing and any thoughts that may be travelling through your mind. Are you comfortable or is the way you have positioned your body causing tension in your back, neck and jaw? Do you wish you could change your posture, but choose not to because where you are reading this paper means that you are expected to sit in a chair in a particular way that is culturally appropriate? Would you rather lie down, but wonder if you did whether you would be frowned upon or would there be a chance you could fall asleep because this is the third paper you have read today.

As a social worker, academic and yoga teacher, I have always been curious about the body and mind and its link to my own and others' well-being. One area of interest has been how the comfort of my own body can impact on how well I do my work and on how I am able to engage with others—especially when it comes to a lack of food, environmental noise or overpowering perfumes (just ask my students!). However, while this body–mind connection has been the subject of conversations with family and friends or I have joked about it in the workplace, I have never had to account for my body in a formal way in relation to any of the family assessments I have conducted; intervention strategies I have chosen to implement; nor when marking students' presentations in the class room. Indeed, from my own experience and student feedback over the years, the academy and many human service workplaces not only ignore the link between the body and mind in theory, but often disregarded it in practice. As the above body scan illustrates, the task of reading an academic paper can be influenced by more than the skill with which the article was written or the relevance of the conceptual knowledge contained within. While this example of the mind–body connection may have somewhat inconsequential outcomes for you the reader and I as the author of this paper, it does highlight the importance of attending to what Ferguson (2009b, p. 474) describes as 'the visceral experience of doing social work' and 'how the senses and emotions impact on perception and workers' and 'service users' capacity to relate to one another'.

According to the Australian Association of Social Workers' (AASW) Education and Accreditation Standards a key goal of social work education is to provide students with opportunities to develop: (1) reflective and reflexive skills; (2) a sound structural analysis; (3) an ability to think critically; and (4) ethical and professional behaviour (AASW, 2000, p. 6). While there is little doubt that social work programmes indeed provide students with such opportunities, anecdotal evidence suggests that most tend to favour a predominantly discursive approach that meets academic standards rather than explore an embodied representation of what these standards may look like in practice. However, as Ferguson (2009b) so aptly points out, in the doing of social work practitioners enter client spaces that evoke deeply tactile and sensual experiences that can thwart practitioners' capacity to implement the standards specified by professional accrediting organisations. Unfortunately, despite the popularity of the person-in-environment approach and some attention to the role of the brain in social work undergraduate degrees, the biological and sociological experience of the body in human activities tends to be ignored. Even though Saleebey noted in 1992 that the quality of both theory and practice had been compromised as a result of the profession's superficial attention to the body, until recently there has been little change in approach (Shapiro and Applegate, 2000; Tangenberg and Kemp, 2002; Cameron and McDermott, 2007).

Cameron and McDermott (2007) suggest that the lack of acknowledgement of the body in social work can be largely attributed to the profession's origins in the post-Enlightenment period. This, they claim, has resulted in an emphasis on developing theoretical and practical interests in a human being with a separate mind and body where the body has faded into obscurity and is rarely problematised. Saleebey (1992) argued, although some years earlier, that the separation of mind and body not only gave rise to the 'technical/rationalist' professions and gave credence to the hegemony of science, but encouraged social work to distance itself from the body in case it legitimised the dominance of the medical model. Even so, recognising that the medical model was as much a political construction as it is epistemological in nature, Saleebey (1992, p. 112) rallied social workers to develop a frame of reference that included 'biological, sensuous, and orgasmic knowledge' infused throughout social work theory and practice to reflect the realities of the profession. However, noting that social work also evolved out of a Western Christian tradition where the body was considered the site of 'sinful desire and private irrationality', Peile (1998) maintained that a major paradigm shift was required before the body would or could be embraced as a valuable source of understanding.

Philosopher Mark Johnson (2007, p. 1) asserts that what we call body and mind are actually 'aspects of one organic process'. Because this concept is at odds with many of our Western traditional philosophical and religious underpinnings *and* our embodied understandings of the words themselves, Johnson suggests that coming to terms with one's own embodiment is one of the most profound philosophical tasks we could ever face. Nevertheless as many neurobiological findings begin to shed light on the interconnectedness between the body, mind and relationship building approaches (Siegel, 2010a, 2010b), some social work scholars are beginning to draw on these to reveal the importance of the body to the profession's understandings rather than needing to challenge the existing dominance of the scientific/medical model (e.g. Applegate and Shapiro, 2005; Lee *et al.*, 2009). By way of example, Cameron and McDermott (2007), in their recent book, draw on both emerging developments in the neuroscientific field as well as sociological understandings of the body to justify moving beyond the Cartesian mind–body divide to present a theoretical base for a practice approach they coin the 'body cognizant social worker'. Drawing attention to the 'corporeal capacity' of both client and worker, Cameron and McDermott (2007, p. 88) suggest that social workers need to explore and ask questions about relevant biological underpinnings between the environment, human affect and learning that may be influencing a particular situation as well as investigate what meaning the body may hold for the client, worker and society.

Using a different theoretical justification but arguably adopting the approach of a 'body cognizant social worker' (Cameron and McDermott, 2007), Ferguson (2009b) has begun to write about the lived experience of practitioners in the field. Taking an interest in an emerging sociological theory, the study of 'mobilities' (Urry, 2007), Ferguson invites us as readers to enter the experience of the child protection worker as they endeavour to meet their statutory obligations while walking, driving and also entering a child and their family's space, system and energies. Infusing his accounts with biological and affective descriptions, Ferguson explores the disorientating experiences of entering these 'intimate' spaces and describes how 'creating order, stillness and gathering yourself so as to perform the core task of remaining child-centred requires a highly skilled performance' (Ferguson, 2009a, p. 475). Ferguson illustrates that writing and thinking about practice in terms of the mobile body contributes to a different theoretical understanding of how a social worker interacts with clients, peers and others in community and how they can also become immobilised and fail to identify issues that may contribute to satisfactory outcomes. Like the observations made during the body scan described above, Ferguson draws attention to how the outcomes of an activity may be influenced as much by the person's experience of the body as by the expectations associated with the situation itself.

Considering the Body in Social Work Education

Reflective practice is thought to be central to effective social work practice and necessary for monitoring worker self-care and well-being (Gibbs, 2001; Knott, 2007). However, recent neuroscientific findings reveal that when people have been traumatised their capacity for reflection and for modulating emotion is largely impaired (Shapiro and Applegate, 2000; van der Kolk, 2006; Forester, 2007). Van der Kolk (2006) states that one of the most compelling findings that neuroimaging of traumatised people's brains has revealed is that under stress, the areas of the brain most needed for 'planning for the future, anticipating the consequences of one's actions, and inhibiting inappropriate responses' are relatively inactive. In fact, for activity to return to the frontal cortex, van der Kolk suggests that the traumatised person must first learn to identify, tolerate and modulate bodily feelings and sensations so as to 'translate their emotions and sensations into a communicable language—understandable, most of all, to themselves' (2006, p. 12). While it may be presumptuous to claim that all social workers are or will be traumatised in their work, there is research to suggest that those drawn to the profession have experienced some disturbing events in their past (Kadushin, 1958; Christie and Kruk, 1998; Coombes and Anderson, 2000; Mensinga, 2010) and that current workers are at greater risk of experiencing Secondary Traumatic Stress and/or compassion fatigue (Valente and Marotta, 2005; Bride and Figley, 2007). In the light of such research, the teaching of the processes for developing and engaging in reflective practice may need to be re-examined.

> As I moved to join one of the small learning groups in my class, I observe how one member of the group is moving uncomfortably in their seat trying hard to remain quiet while the others are silent and withdrawn, determined to resist the inevitable "must" to fill the looming silence created by the task at hand. I become conscious of my own body and wonder if the students are aware of theirs or whether they are so immersed in the academic culture of "disconnect" that, as they spot me walking towards them, they only anticipate what I will ask them about the content of their discussion.
>
> The students' bodily dis-ease reminds me of the unsteadiness that many of the participants in my yoga class experience when they are experimenting with a new posture. When I see the students "fighting" with their body to keep steady while balancing in the tree pose, I draw their attention to their mind and ask them to focus on a spot on the floor or wall in front of them while increasing the length of their exhalation. Yoga teaches that there is a connection between the body, mind and breath and I marvel at how quickly the unsteadiness ceases as the students increase their awareness of all three enabling them to balance with little effort. In this class however, I intended to draw the students' attention to what was happening in their body.
>
> When I enter the group's space, some of the students begin to scribble on their notepads in front of them while others fidget and smile confidently. Rather than ask them about where they are up to in completing the task, I ask each group member to give me a feeling word about what they are experiencing at the present moment. The first student blurts out "I'm not doing all the work this time". Rather than take up the issue presented to me I ask once again for a feeling word. The student stops, her eyes roll to the ceiling, and after a deep inhalation she exhales the word "angry". I nod and shift my gaze to the student next to her and ask him for a feeling word. Looking a bit disarmed, the student seems to hold his breath, fidgets then whispers "confused". Slowly each student names a feeling and, as they do so, something changes in each of their bodies. I draw the students' attention to this change and ask them if they had observed the same thing and to offer me a suggestion as to why this may be so. (Mensinga, 2008–2010)

In the classroom example described above, I begin a process of developing simple conscious awareness (Kondrat, 1999) by bringing the students' attention back into their body in an effort to explore their existing somatic map (Damasio, 1999) and to ponder on how this interacts with their participation in the group exercise. The process of drawing the students' attention to their feelings not only highlights the importance of paying attention to group processes as well as a task, something that social workers understand is critical to successful group work (Johnson and Johnson, 2008), but it provides them with the space in which they can explore their emotional and embodied experiences. Pagis (2009) notes that our embodied responses are based on previous experiences and that embodied self-reflexivity is necessary to change many habitual responses. Drawing on the work of the neuroscientist Damasio (1999), Pagis describes how our body through our nervous system continually monitors our environment (both real and imaginary) in an attempt to maintain some stability within our being. Via this monitoring process, the body produces a map based on sensations unconsciously generated by the body in any given situation which is then transmitted by a non-verbal message about the relationship between it and the objects/environment at any subsequent time. In other words our somatic map, comprising of body sensations that carry instilled meanings about sights, smells, noises, touches etc., must always be navigated even when experiencing an event for the first time.

Coupled with Pagis's (2009) observation that embodied self-reflexivity is necessary to change many habitual responses, Siegel (2010a) highlights the importance of interpersonal 'attunement' for a sense of well-being and a growth towards resiliency within the worker. Also drawing on neuroscientific evidence, Siegel cites the work of Iacoboni (2008) and his work on the role of mirror neurones in experiencing empathy, where one becomes aware of and then replicates the internal state of another. 'Attunement', Siegel (2010a, pp. 41–42) states, involves a process where the worker's mind/body first perceives and engages with the signals emitted by another (initial perception), then embeds the information into their own nervous system (a sub-cortical shift) before assessing the changes in the nervous system (interoception) and then attributing these to the other—a process of simulating the internal state of the other. While social workers like other helping professionals have long recognised the importance of an empathic relationship to the helping process (O'Connor *et al.*, 2003; Beddoe and Maidment, 2009), Iacoboni's (2008) research demonstrates the importance for the worker to be able to tune into their own internal state so they can consciously monitor their response in the presence of the other's experiences—i.e. being open and less reactive, but also cognisant of their own well-being. While there may be concerns and misgivings that a focus on the body may bring with it the risk of a more individualised focus than on relational and power structures, it appears that becoming familiar with our own somatic map is a necessary 'tool' that facilitates future practitioners corporeal capacity to both monitor their reactions as they 'do social work' in client's homes (Ferguson, 2009b) so as to be more proactive than reactive in their decision making and to detect any adverse effects on their personal well-being.

Why Tie the Body in Knots in Social Work Education

About a couple of months ago I was sitting in a meeting and I realised that my legs were completely tied up, crossed, underneath the table, like ... unbelievable! I noticed I was feeling very tense and had to remind myself "you're just sitting in a meeting!". I got myself to uncross my legs and put them down on the floor, but 10 minutes later I found myself in exactly the same position. This time I just thought "wow! I do this all the time". Even though I knew there was no physical danger, my body seemed to be telling me "well yes there is". It was then that I realised that my mind was coming up with all these ideas like "you know you're not supported" and "they don't really want you" and I also found myself becoming all oppositional saying to myself things like "it's me against them". It felt like I was living in my own world and I noticed that I wasn't sure which story was true. Since then I've been wondering why am I prone to this, you know, prone to kind of being, hyper vigilant or anxious or whatever?

That's the question I've taken with me on to the yoga mat and in the last month I've worked out that "oh of course, if you train yourself like that, this is what the outcome is". "Ah! OK! That makes sense to me."

You see I've been an athlete for most of my life. I must have started running at about the age of nine. Back then I used a different body to prepare myself for a race. I would purposely turn on my sympathetic nervous system and just "hype! hype! hype! hype! hype!". I would get myself really nervous, not nervous so that I was out of control, but nervous so that I had this energy, this inner energy that I just had to do something with. I knew when I was ready for the race because I used to get the runs. I'd perfected the technique over the years. As long as I had diarrhoea the day before the race, I knew that I was ready for the race and found that I would do really well. That was great while I was doing athletics and even though I didn't train as much as anybody else, I seemed to be able to do it, you know, just compete. But it's been absolutely awful in my job, in my profession, it just doesn't translate across. I know all about the hyping up and have developed this sympathetic nervous system that works on a hairline trigger but, I don't get to do the running.

Now when I get in situations and I perceive them as dangerous I know that while my body may experience it as that and that my mind will make up stories to try and make sense of the feeling, I can choose what story I want to run with or whether it would even be helpful to run with any. I guess I just have a bit more choice now. (Sue, social worker interviewed August 2010)

Pagis (2009) and Lee *et al.* (2009) claim that practices such as meditation, yoga and other forms of exercise can facilitate awareness of body sensations and an individual's relationship to themselves. However, somewhat akin to choosing whether to react to an itch on the skin or not, yoga practitioners understand that the more familiar they are with their own body and embodied responses, the more likely they are to make an informed choice as to how to react in any given situation. While social work as a profession favours language and communication as the means for self-reflexivity, Sue's description of her body sensations and subsequent understandings illustrates how the body itself can be used as an important anchor for self-knowledge. Sue's experience as an athlete had already given her considerable insight into how to utilise her body to ensure she could run a good race, but it was not until she explored her somatic map on the yoga mat that Sue realised that her preparation regime was now negatively impacting on her day-to-day experience as a social worker. Once making the link, Sue was better able to decide on how to enlist her body in the workplace rather than remain reactive.

Yoga has gained increasing popularity in the Western world (van der Kolk, 2006; Penman *et al.*, 2008). Although some scholars are questioning the philosophical origins of modern yoga as it is practised today (Alter, 2004; Singleton, 2010), due to its increasing popularity in the general population it may be timely to include Hatha Yoga as a mindfulness awareness practice to facilitate both embodied reflective practice in social work education and professional practice. Kabat-Zin (2004), the founder of the Mindfulness Based Stress Reduction (MBSR) programme, includes yoga as part of the curriculum. He notes that Hatha Yoga can be done as a slow meditative practice as well as a preferred way for those who find sitting and/or meditation difficult. Interestingly, while the practices of Hatha Yoga and meditation tend to be seen as separate today and are typically researched as such, traditionally they have always been linked. In his Sutras describing the Eightfold path of Yoga, Patanjali described the postures and meditation as two separate limbs, but noted that they are intertwined. As Faulds (2008, p. 95) so nicely states: 'Yoga and meditation are complementary practices. Yoga brings you to the meditation cushion relaxed and present. Meditation deepens your capacity for self awareness, making your time on the yoga mat more mindful'.

Mindfulness and its contribution to client and human service workers' well-being has been explored more extensively in recent years—including in social work practice and education (e.g. Birnbaum, 2008; Lynn, 2009). However, just as the body is veiled in much of the social work literature, few studies explore what yoga can add as a Mindful Awareness Practice (Shapiro and Carlson, 2009). Lynn (2009), drawing on a spiritual paradigm rather than a neurobiological one, notes that mindfulness and mindfulness meditation can be used as effective tools for developing self-observation and awareness in the learning process. Although Lynn identifies scanning body sensations and focusing on the breath as techniques in developing mindfulness, the role of the body is not explored to any great extent. Pagis (2009), by way of contrast, uses neurobiological explanations to discuss the success of body scan techniques to increase embodied self-reflexivity. As was noted previously in this paper, Pagis draws on Damasio (1999) to highlight the effectiveness of the technique to raise awareness of an individual's somatic map to facilitate new forms of self-anchoring. In keeping with this perspective, yoga teacher and psychotherapist Stone (2010, p. 207) claims that the yoga masters didn't so much practise yoga as a form of exercise but rather as an opportunity to map the energetic pathways of the body.

Although little research has been done in relation to the health benefits yoga can offer social workers and students alike, from my own personal experience and that of others (for example, Sue, as above), becoming aware of visceral experiences and somatic messages appears to provide much needed information for practice and facilitates greater awareness for personal well-being. In a small study exploring psychotherapists' (two were social workers) experience of engaging in a regular yoga practice, Valente and Marotta (2005) identified a number of benefits, including:

1. Yoga increased participants' 'awareness not only of what their bodies were feeling and communicating but also their thoughts, emotions and patterns of cognition' (2005, p. 72). They noted that this developing awareness was useful as a technique to develop emotional regulation and helped them gauge their stress levels.
2. Yoga provided participants with the opportunity to achieve better balance in their lives and avoid burnout. They noted that they were better able to 'calm their central

nervous system, reduce anxiety, reduce mental stress and fatigue, helped them to relax and gave them overall feelings of being "centred and grounded"' (2005, p. 74).

3. Yoga became a 'way of life' that helped them become calmer, more mentally and emotionally stabile and led to personal growth (2005, p. 77).

Drawing on their experience of running yoga classes for people who have experienced trauma, Emerson *et al.* (2009b) claim that yoga offers the participant an opportunity to notice the body, make friends with it and draw on it as a resource in a relative place of safety. As previously stated, many students need more introductory experiences before critical reflective essays, process recordings and gestalt techniques can be utilised to develop reflective capacity. Moreover, given some of those drawn to social work as a profession have experienced traumatising events in their past and could find reflection a difficult task to engage in, if not re-traumatising, attention to 'healing' somatic maps is essential. Although it has been argued that any form of body 'work out' can facilitate embodied self-reflexivity (Pagis, 2009), recognition of the mind–body connection is necessary to develop mindful awareness. Yoga and other Eastern embodied practices are predicated on this assumption and because of their increasing acceptance in the general community their accessibility is assured and can be used as an adjunct to social work education. Emerson and his colleagues (Emerson *et al.*, 2009a) note that yoga classes can be especially effective because they are conducted in a group situation and offer participants the chance to practise among other things: being in the present moment; making choices by deciding how to do a particular posture; and taking effective action if and when they experience any discomfort during a class.

Conclusion

The introduction of embodied practices like yoga will no doubt challenge the mind–body split that is prevalent not only in the profession but also in education institutions today. However, given the importance of reflection and self-awareness in social work and increasing evidence that when the body's somatic map is ignored or misunderstood it can supersede critical thinking and impede reflective practice (Rothschild, 2000; Ogden *et al.*, 2006; van der Kolk, 2006; Forester, 2007; Siegel, 2010b), it is time for the profession to consider the affective nature of embodied struggles, particularly in the academy. In his book, *Full Catastrophe Living*, Kabat-Zinn expresses surprise at how as a society we can be 'simultaneously completely preoccupied with the appearance of our own body and at the same time completely out of touch with it' (2004, p. 75). Of course this phenomenon has been explored and theorised by sociologists and feminists alike who note that the body image 'is as much a function of the subject's psychology and sociohistorical context as anatomy' (Grosz, 1994, p. 79). While Kabat-Zinn expresses his surprise to draw attention to how *experiencing* the body without the overlay of judgement can change an individual's view of it and enable them to better monitor and deal with stress, pain and illness, the point raised by Grosz (1994) brings our attention back to the call to *reposition* the body within the social work profession (Saleebey, 1992; Peile, 1998; Lee *et al.*, 2009).

While I recognise that including embodied practices in an already overcrowded academic curriculum maybe challenging, I also believe that merely acknowledging the role of the body as an important source of knowledge may begin a process of exploration that currently does not exist. As Cameron and McDermott (2007, p. 92) note, acknowledging the importance of the body in social work theory and practice is necessary not only in relation to client outcomes but is also essential to ensure the well-being of the social worker and to account for themselves 'as an embodied actor entering and engaging with the client's world'.

References

Alter, J. S. (2004) *Yoga in Modern India: The Body between Science and Philosophy*, Princeton University Press, Princeton, NJ.

Applegate, J. S. & Shapiro, J. R. (2005) *Neurobiology for Clinical Social Work: Theory and Practice*, W.W. Norton & Company, New York.

Australian Association of Social Workers (AASW) (2000) *National Practice Standards of the Australian Association of Social Workers* [online]. Available at: http://www.aasw.asn.au/, accessed 2 February 2010.

Badger, K., Royse, D. & Craig, C. (2008) 'Hospital social workers and indirect trauma exposure: an exploratory study of contributing factors', *Health and Social Work*, vol. 33, no. 1, pp. 63–71.

Beddoe, L. & Maidment, J. (2009) *Mapping Knowledge for Social Work Practice*, Cengage Learning Australia, Melbourne.

Birnbaum, L. (2008) 'The use of mindfulness training to create an "accompanying place" for social work students', *Social Work Education: The International Journal*, vol. 27, no. 8, pp. 837–852.

Bresler, L. (ed.) (2004) *Knowing Bodies, Moving Minds: Towards Embodied Teaching and Learning*, Kluwer Academic Publishers, Boston, MA.

Bride, B. E. & Figley, C. R. (2007) 'The fatigue of compassionate social workers: an introduction to the special issue on compassion fatigue', *Clinical Social Work Journal*, vol. 35, pp. 151–153.

Cameron, N. & McDermott, F. (2007) *Social Work & the Body*, Palgrave MacMillan, Houndmills, Basingstoke.

Christie, A. & Kruk, E. (1998) 'Choosing to become a social worker: motives, incentives, concerns and disincentives', *Social Work Education*, vol. 17, no. 1, pp. 21–34.

Coombes, K. & Anderson, R. (2000) 'The impact of family of origin on social workers from alcoholic families', *Clinical Social Work Journal*, vol. 28, no. 3, pp. 281–302.

Crossley, N. (2001) 'Embodiment and social structure: a response to Howson and Inglis', *The Sociological Review*, vol. 49, no. 3, pp. 318–326.

Damasio, A. (1999) *The Feeling of What Happens: Body and Emotion in the Making of Consciousness*, University of California Press, San Diego, CA.

Emerson, D., Sharma, R., Chaudhry, S. & Turner, J. (2009a) 'Trauma-sensitive yoga: principles, practice, and research', *International Journal of Yoga Therapy*, vol. 19, pp. 123–128.

Emerson, D., Turner, J. & van der Kolk, B. (2009b) 'Toward becoming a trauma-sensitive yoga teacher', *Trauma-Sensitive Yoga Instruction: A Teacher's Certificate Training (November 8–12, 2009)*, Kripalu Yoga Centre, The Trauma Centre at JRI Lennox, Massachusetts.

Faulds, R. (2008) 'Yoga: bringing together body and mind', in *Quietmind: A Beginner's Guide to Meditation*, ed. S. Piver, Shambhala, Boston, MA, pp. 94–101.

Ferguson, H. (2009a) 'Driven to care: the car, automobility and social work', *Mobilities*, vol. 4, no. 2, pp. 275–290.

Ferguson, H. (2009b) 'Performing child protection: home visiting, movement and the struggle to reach the abused child', *Child & Family Social Work*, vol. 14, no. 4, pp. 471–480.

Forester, C. (2007) 'Your own body of wisdom: recognising and working with somatic transference with dissociative and traumatised patients', *Body, Movement and Dance in Psychotherapy*, vol. 2, no. 2, pp. 123–133.

Gibbs, J. A. (2001) 'Maintaining front-line workers in child protection: a case for refocusing supervision', *Child Abuse Review*, vol. 10, no. 5, pp. 323–335.

Goleman, D. (2006) *Social Intelligence: The New Science of Human Relationships*, Bantam Books, New York.

Grosz, E. (1994) *Volatile Bodies: Toward a Corporeal Feminism*, Allen & Unwin, St Leonards.

Howson, A. & Inglis, D. (2001) 'The body in sociology: tension inside and outside sociological thought', *The Sociological Review*, vol. 49, no. 3, pp. 297–317.

Iacoboni, M. (2008) *Mirroring People*, Farrar, Straus and Girroux, New York.

Johnson, D. R. & Johnson, F. P. (2008) *Joining Together: Group Theory and Group Skills*. 10th edn. Allyn and Bacon, Boston, MA.

Johnson, M. (2007) *The Meaning of the Body: Aesthetics of Human Understanding*, The University of Chicago Press, Chicago, IL.

Kabat-Zinn, J. (2004) *Full Catastrophe Living: How to Cope with Stress, Pain and Illness Using Mindfulness Meditation*. 15th Anniversary edn. Piatkus Books, London.

Kadushin, A. (1958) 'Determinants of career choice and their implications for social work', *Social Work Education*, vol. 6, pp. 17–21.

Knott, C. (2007) 'Reflective practice revisited', in *Reflective Practice in Social Work*, eds C. Knott & T. Scragg, Learning Matters, Exeter.

Kondrat, M. E. (1999) 'Who is the "self" in self aware: professional self awareness from a critical theory perspective', *Social Service Review*, vol. 73, no. 4, pp. 451–477.

Koritsas, S., Coles, J. & Boyle, M. (2010) 'Workplace violence towards social workers: the Australian experience', *British Journal of Social Work*, vol. 40, no. 1, pp. 257–271.

Lee, M. Y., Ng, S. M., Leung, P. P. Y. & Chan, C. L. W. (2009) *Integrative Body–Mind–Spirit Social Work: An Empirically Based Approach to Assessment and Treatment*, Oxford University Press, USA.

Lynn, R. (2009) 'Mindfulness in social work education', *Social Work Education: The International Journal*, vol. 29, no. 3, pp. 289–304.

Markula, P. (2004) 'Embodied movement knowledge in fitness and exercise education', in *Knowing Bodies, Moving Minds*, ed. L. Bresler, Kluwer Academic Publishers, Dordrecht, pp. 61–76.

Mensinga, J. (2008–2010) *Personal Journal Notes*, James Cook University, Cairns.

Mensinga, J. (2010) *Quilting Professional Stories: A Gendered Experience of Choosing Social Work as a Career*, VDM Verlag Dr Müller, Saarbrücken.

O'Connor, I., Wilson, J. & Setterlund, D. (2003) *Social Work and Welfare*. 4th edn. Pearson Education Australia, Frenchs Forest.

Ogden, P., Minton, K. & Pain, C. (2006) *Trauma and the Body: A Sensorimotor Approach to Psychotherapy*, W.W. Norton & Company, New York.

Pagis, M. (2009) 'Embodied self-reflexivity', *Social Psychology Quarterly*, vol. 72, pp. 265–283.

Peile, C. (1998) 'Emotional and embodied knowledge: implications for critical practice', *Journal of Sociology and Social Welfare*, vol. 25, no. 4, pp. 39–59.

Penman, S., Cohen, M., Stevens, P. & Jackson, S. (2008) *Yoga in Australia: Results of a National Survey*, RMIT University, Melbourne.

Pryce, J. G., Shackleford, K. K. & Pryce, D. H. (2007) *Secondary Traumatic Stress and the Child Welfare Professional*, Lyceum Books, Inc, Chicago, IL.

Rothschild, B. (2000) *The Body Remembers: The Psychophysiology of Trauma and Trauma Treatment*, W.W. Norton & Company, New York.

Saleebey, D. (1992) 'Biology's challenge to social work: embodying the person-in-environment perspective', *Social Work*, vol. 37, no. 2, pp. 112–118.

Satterfield, J. (2010) 'A twisted story', in *Freeing the Body Freeing the Mind: Writings on the Connections between Yoga and Buddhism*, ed. M. Stone, Shambhala, Boston, MA.

Shapiro, J. R. & Applegate, J. S. (2000) 'Cognitive neuroscience, neurobiology and affect regulation: implications for clinical social work', *Clinical Social Work Journal*, vol. 28, no. 1, pp. 9–21.

Shapiro, S. L. & Carlson, L. E. (2009) *The Art and Science of Mindfulness: Integrating Mindfulness into Psychology and the Helping Professions*, American Psychological Association, Washington, DC.

Siegel, D. J. (2010a) *The Mindful Therapist: A Clinician's Guide to Mindsight and Neural Integration*, W.W. Norton & Company, New York.

Siegel, D. J. (2010b) *Mindsight: The New Science of Personal Transformation*, Bantam Books, New York.

Singleton, M. (2010) *Yoga Body: The Origins of Modern Posture Practice*, Oxford University Press, New York.

Stanley, J. & Goddard, C. (2002) *In the Firing Line: Power and Violence in Child Protection Work*, Wiley, London.

Stone, M. (2010) *Freeing the Body Freeing the Mind: Writings on the Connections between Yoga and Buddhism*, Shambhala, Boston, MA.

Tangenberg, K. M. & Kemp, S. (2002) 'Embodied practice: claiming the body's experience, agency, and knowledge for social work', *Social Work*, vol. 47, pp. 9–18.

Urry, J. (2007) *Mobilities*, Polity, Cambridge, MA.

Valente, V. & Marotta, A. (2005) 'The impact of yoga on the professional and personal life of the psychotherapist', *Contemporary Family Therapy*, vol. 27, no. 1, pp. 65–79.

van der Kolk, B. (1994) 'The body keeps the score: memory & the evolving psychobiology of post traumatic stress', *Harvard Review of Psychiatry*, vol. 1, no. 5, pp. 253–265.

van der Kolk, B. (2006) 'Clinical implications of neuroscience research in PTSD', *Annals of the New York Academy of Sciences*, vol. 1071, pp. 277–293.

If a Holistic Approach to Social Work Requires Acknowledgement of Religion, What Does This Mean for Social Work Education?

Beth R. Crisp

There is growing recognition that promoting wellbeing requires a holistic approach to social work practice which includes understanding the role of religion in the lives of service users. This is reflected in a number of mentions of religion in the new code of ethics produced by the Australian Association of Social Workers. However, any consideration of whether religion has a place in social work should not only occur at the individual level, but also consider faith-based agencies. This paper considers the implications of this for social work education in respect of developing curriculum which acknowledges the religious dimension of the lives of many service users; skill development to enable social workers to broach issues of religion with service users; and working in or with faith-based agencies.

Introduction

Social work has long prided itself on being a holistic profession interested in both the person and their environment, and considers a range of individual and contextual factors as contributing to wellbeing. As such, in addition to being concerned with ensuring essential resources for maintaining or regaining physical and mental health, as well as social and other opportunities, in recent years there has been a growing awareness of the necessity for social work practitioners to take account of the spiritual needs of service users (e.g. Canda and Furman, 1999; Lindsay, 2002; Nash and Stewart, 2002; Gale *et al.*, 2007; Mathews, 2009; Crisp, 2010a; Holloway and Moss, 2010). While there are many people who use the terms 'spirituality' and 'religion' interchangeably and for whom their spirituality is how they live out their religious beliefs, there are others who have argued that one can be spiritual but not religious (e.g. Ai, 2002; Adams *et al.*, 2008; Holloway and Moss, 2010). Hence it has been suggested that 'Religion is a personal or institutionalized system grounded in a set of beliefs, values and practices. In contrast, spirituality ... is a personal state or manner of being' (Barnett *et al.*, 2000, p. 574) which may or may not reflect religious beliefs. Moreover, it has been claimed that for many people spirituality is a far more preferable concept than religion:

> A few people see very little difference between religion and spirituality. Most make a clear distinction. Religion tends to be associated with what is publicly available, such as churches, mosques, Bibles, prayer books, religious officials, weddings and funerals. It also regularly includes uncomfortable associations with boredom, narrow-mindedness and being out of date, as well as more disconcerting links with fanaticism, bigotry, cruelty and persecution. It seems that in many people's minds religion is firmly caught up in the cold brutalities of history.
>
> Spirituality is almost always seen as much warmer, associated with love, inspiration, wholeness, depth, mystery and personal devotions like prayer and meditation. (Hay and Nye, 2006, p. 19)

While not necessarily for the reasons outlined by Hay and Nye, there has nevertheless been a history of ambivalence towards religion within professional social work in countries such as Australia (see Crisp, 2010a, 2010b). It has thus been pleasing to see a small number of books emerging in recent years from British social work academics which have focused more specifically on issues associated with religion in social work practice (e.g. Moss, 2005; Ashencaen Crabtree *et al.*, 2008; Furness and Gilligan, 2010) as there has been a tendency to ignore religion unless it is somewhat exotic or problematic, and even then it tends to be considered as an issue in which cultural competence is required rather than understanding a person's religion as a potential resource (cf. Furness and Gilligan, 2010). This is despite a growing body of literature which suggests that religious beliefs and practices can lead to enhanced wellbeing for some individuals and communities [for a summary of this literature see Lee and Newberg (2005)]. Furthermore, despite the fact that being a person of religious beliefs is one of the most common reasons for persecution (Hodge, 2007), the promotion of religious freedom has not been a priority within the profession even though social workers are expected to ensure that human rights for all are promoted. Moreover, it has been claimed that failing to address religious dimensions results in unethical practice (Amato-von Hemert, 1994; Hodge, 2005) and legislative imperatives that human service providers take account of the religious and spiritual needs of service users are emerging in some countries (Moss, 2005).

In this paper I will be focusing particularly on the place of religion in social work practice and social work education rather than the relationship between spirituality and social work which, as previously indicated, has been covered by several authors in recent years. My interest in considering this topic arose out of my reading of two recent publications. The first was *Religion, Belief and Social Work: Making a Difference* by British authors Sheila Furness and Philip Gilligan (2010). This book included a thought-provoking reflection by a social work manager who noted that the question of religion was never noted despite being one of the elements in the assessment framework which they were using. In raising this with a colleague she was told 'You know, unless a family is really strictly Muslim and it's obvious, the social workers aren't even asking, they're not even looking at it as a topic' (in Furness and Gilligan, 2010, p. 36). After raising this issue with other staff, it was clear that they were uncomfortable discussing religion with service users:

> My social workers said, "Can we ask that?". I think that they thought that it was too intrusive to ask somebody about religion, but I said, "We talk about relationships, mum and dad, what kind of relationship do they have, do they have time together, do they have time as a couple? So if we're talking about really personal things, I think we're going to be okay if we ask them about religion". (In Furness and Gilligan, 2010, p. 37)

In Australia, where there is no state church, social workers sometimes call on notions such as the separation of church and state as justification for not discussing issues of religion with service users, particularly if their positions are government funded. Yet despite the existence of a state church and mandated questions about religion in widely used assessment frameworks, it would seem that English social workers are also reluctant to discuss issues of religion with service users.

While thinking about this question of whether social workers, including myself, found it easier to discuss many very personal issues but not religion, I found that in the 2010 revisions to its *Code of Ethics*, the Australian Association of Social Workers (AASW) made far more references to religion than in its predecessor (AASW, 1999). In the previous code of ethics these were requirements to prevent discrimination on the basis of religion, the need for social workers to remain aware of conflicts of interest on the basis of religion and the need to be aware of their own religious values (AASW, 1999). While these remain, there are a number of additional areas in which religion is now being discussed including two clauses under the broad heading of 'Respect for human dignity and worth':

> Social workers will respect others' beliefs, religious or spiritual world-views, values, culture, goals, needs and desires, as well as kinship and communal bonds, within a framework of social justice and human rights. (AASW, 2010, p. 17)

One manifestation of this respect is how social workers engage with religious individuals or organisations. Hence under a 'Commitment to practice competence' it has been proposed that:

> When engaged in social work interventions that are influenced by their spiritual or religious world views, social workers will ensure that they do so in a competent, transparent and accountable manner, in accordance with the ethical standards outlined in this *Code*. (AASW, 2010, p. 22)

The questions which are being considered in the remainder of this paper concerning whether there is a place for religion in social work, the role of faith-based agencies and implications for social work education, first emerged from my reflections as an Australian social work educator. However, these appear to be questions which are being considered by social workers in a number of countries and what follows is an attempt to answer these questions using the international literature.

Is There a Place for Religion in Social Work?

The inclusion of references to religion in the AASW's new code of ethics seemingly presuppose that there is a place for religion in social work. However, in both Australia and elsewhere, this has been a topic for debate among social workers. Reservations about there being a place for religion in social work are frequently around religious values, and in particular where social work theory and values are dissimilar from religious ideals (Bowpitt, 2000). As Peter Gilbert, an English social worker has noted:

> We are deeply ambivalent about religious groupings; when faith communities care for their own and dress respectfully, we laud their sense of civic responsibility; when difference becomes too acute, we accuse them of not integrating, and failing to become more "like us"—whatever that means. (Gilbert, 2007, p. 20)

Concerns about the involvement of religious organisations in social work provision have often been based on fears that vulnerable service users could readily be preyed on by workers driven more by religious zeal than the values of social work. There may be questions about whether staff have been hired more on the basis of their religious beliefs than their professional skills or knowledge and there may be justifiable fears of service users being discriminated against if they resist participation in activities with an explicitly religious focus (Tangenberg, 2005).

Religious viewpoints which have been aligned with oppressive practices, and which have reinforced, rather than challenged, social exclusion, further contributed to negative beliefs about religion among social workers (Moss, 2005). It is sometimes claimed that welfare reforms have at times been eroded by governments under pressure from right wing, conservative and often religious lobby groups (Vanderwoerd, 2006). Indeed religious discourses are often uncritically promoted within social work as being anti-women's rights, unsupportive of women who wish to leave violent relationships, and associated with extreme religious militias, as well as unsupportive of programmes to alleviate poverty (Hodge, 2002). While such allegations may apply to some religious groups and organisations, there are also many organisations with a religious auspice which promote gender equality, run effective anti-poverty programmes and support women who do seek to move away from living in violent circumstances. Furthermore, there is a growing realisation that there are synergies between social work theory and some understandings of religion and spirituality (Dezerotes, 2006).

Although it is possible to intellectually recognise points of convergence between religious values and social work theory and practice, individuals may choose to keep apart those aspects of their lives which they consider personal (i.e. religious beliefs) from their public or professional lives. This applies not only to service users but also to social workers who may have experienced undermining of their professional credibility by colleagues who consider any expression of religious beliefs as evidence of some form of psychopathology or resulted in suggestions that they are fundamentalists and unable to practise social work in an anti-oppressive manner (Gilligan, 2003). In some agencies, forbidding social workers from revealing anything of their religion goes beyond discussing their beliefs, to bans on clothing or jewellery which have religious symbolism. Hence it is with some interest that the recent draft of a new code of ethics for the Australian Association of Social Workers (AASW) states that

> In carrying out their professional practice responsibilities, social workers are entitled to reciprocal rights, which include the right to ... hold cultural, religious or spiritual world views and for these to be acknowledged in the workplace and professional contexts to the extent that they do not impinge on the other guidelines in this *Code*. (AASW, 2010, p. 16)

Being afforded respect for their own religious and spiritual beliefs won't necessarily lead to a difference in how social workers practise. For example, although one survey of 123 graduate social work students in a public Midwestern US university revealed that more than four-fifths (82.9%) agreed that their spirituality was relevant in their professional lives, this didn't necessarily translate into their work with service users and very few claim they would encourage a service user to join or leave a religion (Rizer and McColley, 1996). Many social workers are conscious of the need to ensure they don't project their own religious beliefs and understandings onto those of service users (Gollnick, 2005) as doing so is likely to be interpreted as disrespecting a service user's rights to self-determination (Wagler-Martin, 2005). Hence actions such as praying with clients are typically deemed to be professionally inappropriate (Doel *et al.*, 2009) although some social workers are known to do this.

The Role of Faith-Based Agencies

In countries like Australia, where church agencies are some of the largest employers of social workers (Camilleri and Winkworth, 2004), any serious consideration of the place of religion in social work leads to the question as to what is the role of faith-based agencies in service provision. The AASW's proposed Code of Ethics specifically notes a requirement for social workers to be respectful of faith-based agencies:

> Social workers will recognise, acknowledge and remain sensitive to and respectful of the religious and spiritual world views of individuals, groups, communities and social networks, and the operations and missions of faith and spiritually-based organisations. (AASW, 2010, p. 18)

Until early in the twentieth century, there were very few welfare services in much of the Western world which were not provided by religious organisations and the theoretical underpinnings of the services they provided tended to be based on interpretations of religious teaching (Bowpitt, 1998; Canda and Furman, 1999; Graham, 2007). Nevertheless, this 'legacy has been the skeleton in the cupboard, something best forgotten and preferably ignored' (Bowpitt, 1998, p. 676). Despite a rapid growth of social work services in non-religious settings, such that in many places social work services are predominantly provided by secular agencies, religious groups continue to play a significant role in the provision of social work services and are entrenched in the system of welfare provision (Vanderwoerd, 2006). For example, even though the major providers of social work services are local authorities, it has been estimated that more than 23,000 religious charitable organisations provide support and services to individual and communities within the United Kingdom (Furness and Gilligan, 2010).

In what are sometimes termed 'faith-based' agencies, many agencies and programmes which are auspiced by churches or religious organisations often run at arms-length from overtly religious aspects of such bodies, and the notion of being a faith-based agency may be questionable (Melville and McDonald, 2006). This is particularly so when the work is largely funded by government, as there is usually some requirement that funded services will be made available to individuals who do not share the religious beliefs of the service provider, and that the funding per se is not for the propagation of the faith. In such agencies, there will not necessarily be any overt religious imagery on view and many of the social workers and other agency staff would not necessarily identify with the religion of their employer. Nevertheless, a religious ethos tends to underpin the broad aims and objectives of agencies with a religious auspice, although this may be termed more like an 'imperative to care' (Moss, 2002, p. 39) than in explicitly religious language.

One way in which this 'imperative to care' is realised in practice is that religious groups have often seen areas of need and established services, particularly to service the needs of the most disadvantaged in the community (Winkworth and Camilleri, 2004). For example, in the late nineteenth century, the Salvation Army is credited as establishing the first labour bureau open to all unemployed Australians as well as the world's first programme for released prisoners (Salvation Army, 2010). The need for such services was eventually recognised by governments who either took over the running of or established their own services in these areas. Moving forward to the twenty-first century, church agencies continue to pioneer new forms of service delivery and are key providers of services to refugees, despite the fact that many refugees entering Australia do not identify with the major religious groupings in Australia.

In addition to being motivated by religious beliefs, it has been proposed that a second characteristic which distinguished faith-based organisations from their secular counterparts is the relationship with a religious constituency or group of stakeholders (Ferris, 2005). These groups have often have provided funding in the form of property, people, and finances over long periods of time and may be satisfied with providing needed services to the community purely on the basis of altruism. However, there may be tensions if some stakeholders believe that faith-based agencies have a right to impart their religious beliefs to service users. While some groups may make deliberate decisions to keep separate their religious and welfare arms, so that the latter might receive government funding (Goździak, 2002), others which work from a more explicit religious basis and have parts of their programmes with a strong religious focus have often opted not to receive public funding which would limit such activities (Tangenberg, 2005).

Implications for Social Work Education

Although *Global Standards for the Education and Training of the Social Work Profession* acknowledges the need for social work education to promote respect for different religions and for social workers to have some knowledge as to the role religion plays in the lives of the service users of social work services (IASSW and IFSW, 2004), teaching about religion tends of be considered optional, or in other words not required, in many schools of social work (Furman *et al.*, 2005). Consequently, the thinking which underpins the proposed changes to the AASW's code of ethics, as well as other recent writings on the interface between religion and social work, potentially poses a number of challenges for social work educators. In particular, I will focus on three key issues:

- curriculum which acknowledges the religious dimension of the lives of many service users;
- skill development to enable social workers to broach issues of religion with service users; and
- working in or with faith-based agencies.

Curriculum

One way of getting religion into the social work curriculum is to invite a university chaplain, or going beyond the university, to invite a hospital chaplain or some prominent religious educator to come and present a lecture or facilitate a workshop on the topic. Exposure to religious professionals can challenge stereotypes which students may have developed in the absence of any actual prior engagement with such individuals. However, not all of us have access to religious professionals who we would want to come and teach social work students. Moreover, some of us have experiences of university chaplains whose demeanour has been an antithesis to the values of tolerance for diversity which underpin our curricula (Tacey, 2003). Furthermore, in order to demonstrate how religion can be integrated into social work practice, there is arguably a strong case for input on religion to be taught by someone from within the profession (Crisp, 2009).

The possibility of having an elective unit focusing on religion and social work has been proposed by some (Sheridan *et al.*, 1994) but a difficulty with this approach is that confining input on religion to an elective is likely to result in only students who already have an interest in religion, and are more likely to be sympathetic to religious ideas, enrolling in such a course of study. Such an approach also fails to recognise how frequently issues associated with religion emerge in social work practice with one study of social workers estimating that around one-third of all service users presented with issues in which religion or spirituality was potentially an issue (Sheridan *et al.*, 1992). This is not surprising if the life events which bring some people into contact with social workers are the same life events which result in some people turning to religion (Ai, 2002). Hence a more authentic way of incorporating religion into the social work curriculum is for it to be one of the many characteristics or aspects of human life which are discussed across the curriculum (Ai, 2002). For example, in my own university we have sought to include exemplars or readings relating to rural social work and social work with indigenous Australians, in several units in our Bachelor of Social Work degree. Arguably a similar approach could be taken with religion, but in doing so, it would be important to ensure that the material was appropriately embedded into the curriculum and not done in a tokenistic way which reinforces unhelpful stereotypes.

For many social work educators, the greatest hurdle in including mentions of religion in the curriculum is arguably our own inhibitions about discussing religion. This not only applies to those who are not religious or have little interest in religion, as reluctance to discuss religion in the professional context can readily be found among those of us who value the role of religion in our own lives (see also Lindsay, 2002; Holloway and Moss, 2010). Living in what has been described as 'a deliberately secular nation' (Breward, 1988, p. 99), it is not easy to discuss religious beliefs and practices without running the risk of wrath from students who are anti-religious, especially those who regard any non-negative mention of religion as some form of proselytising. Nor is it easy to discuss how religion can play a positive role in some people's lives at a time when religious institutions are regularly in the news due to scandals such as abuse of children or when it is claimed that terrorist acts have been associated with fanatical or fundamentalist religious beliefs.

While not including discussion of matters associated with religion which might be more comfortable for many social work educators (Sheridan *et al.*, 1994), issues such as promoting respect for religious beliefs other than one's own, or understanding the place of religion in the lives of service users, risk being neglected in the curriculum.

Skill Development

It has been proposed that 'service users need opportunities to discuss their religious and spiritual beliefs, and the strengths, difficulties and needs that arise from them' (Furness and Gilligan, 2010, p. 44) in environments where they will not feel judged for the holding of religious or spiritual beliefs, particularly if these beliefs are not widely held in the community. Religious beliefs and practices can have many different functions, including facilitating connectedness, establishing a sense of identity, providing structures for quiet reflection, finding a sense of meaning or experiencing transcendence (Crisp, 2010a). Hence for social workers, knowing what an individual obtains or is seeking from their religion may be more important information than what a person's religious beliefs are. In other words,

> Rather than beginning by asking "what is wrong with this person", we begin our questioning from a different perspective and ask different questions: "What gives this person's life meaning?", "What is it that keeps them going, even in the midst of their psychological pain and turmoil?", "Where is this person's primary source of value?", "What can be done to enhance their being?". In asking such questions, the person's situation is reframed in a way that reveals hidden dimensions. (Swinton, 2001, p. 138)

Of course, there are many service users for whom religion is of no importance or of very limited importance, and in making a space in which people are enabled to discuss religion, also provide a sense of permission which allows them to decline speaking of this aspect of their lives. Nevertheless, a holistic assessment requires some understanding of what really matters to people. While there are some situations in which social workers can get by with very limited information about service users and not compromise the service given, there are many situations when we should attempt to take account of what really matters for people. As one Canadian social worker suggests:

> I say, I'm really interested in understanding what this means for you. And is there anything about your own cultural background, or what this means in your own community, that would be helpful for me to understand, because I may not know that. I'm not going to assume anything ... I'm going to wait and hear how it's been constructed in their lives. (In Clark, 2006)

Working in this way provides social workers with opportunities to open up discussion of issues, such as particular religions or religious practices, which they have limited or no knowledge of rather than demanding the social worker have expert knowledge. Whether or not such conversations result in explicit discussions about religion, any discussion about what is meaningful in people's lives will require social workers to have the skills and sensitivity needed to appropriately respond to issues which emerge. However, arguably this is a skill which a competent social worker has, whatever setting they are working in.

Working with Faith-Based Agencies

Although faith-based agencies are major providers of welfare services, this form of agency receives little or no mention in contemporary textbooks in the area of human service agencies (e.g. Hafford-Letchfield, 2009). While it could be debated whether or not students need specific input on faith-based agencies as part of their social work education, they nevertheless do need to be able to work effectively with organisations in which the aims, values and structures have arisen from a philosophical and value basis other than social work (Gardner, 2006). This may require working with other professions and/or volunteers (Angell, 2010). Even if not employed in faith-based agencies themselves, social workers must often interact with these agencies, particularly when universal provision of welfare services provided by the welfare state is lacking and faith-based agencies step in to fill residual needs (Edgardh and Pettersson, 2010; Pessi, 2010).

Social workers employed by faith-based agencies may observe or experience a number of tensions and need the analytical skills to determine their stance on these issues. These include whether the role of a faith-based agency is primarily to be a state-funded welfare agency or a critical voice speaking out on behalf of the most disadvantaged members of the society (Angell, 2010). While the former may allow for social work values to predominate, e.g. a faith-based foster care agency approving same-sex couples to act as foster parents despite the religious teachings of the agency's auspicing body (Furness and Gilligan, 2010), it can also lead to the silencing of criticisms against the state (Valasik, 2010). In faith-based agencies which have operated as *de facto* arms of the welfare state, there may be tensions if agencies are exploring ways in which the religious and spiritual values of the agency can be made more explicit (Crisp, 2010a). Finally, working in a faith-based agency may challenge any division between one's personal religious beliefs and one's professional practice (Furness and Gilligan, 2010).

Conclusion

This paper has proposed a case as to why promoting wellbeing requires a holistic approach to social work which includes an acknowledgement both of the role of religion in the lives of service users and the contribution of faith-based agencies to service provision, and considered the implications of this for social work education. The prevailing religious climate and predominant religions within a society, as well as the role of faith-based agencies in service provision, should undoubtedly influence how this occurs. There are no definitive blueprints but readers are nevertheless encouraged to consider if and how they currently incorporate religion into the social work curriculum and whether this is adequate.

References

Adams, K., Hyde, B. & Woolley, R. (2008) *The Spiritual Dimension of Childhood*, Jessica Kingsley Publishers, London.

Ai, A. L. (2002) 'Integrating spirituality into professional education: a challenging but feasible task', *Journal of Teaching in Social Work*, vol. 22, pp. 103–130.

Amato-von Hemert, K. (1994) 'Should social work education address religious issues? Yes!', *Journal of Social Work Education*, vol. 30, pp. 7–11.

Angell, O. H. (2010) 'Sacred welfare agents in secular welfare states: the Church of Norway in Drammen', in *Welfare and Religion in 21st Century Europe: Volume 1. Configuring the Connections*, eds A. Bäckström, G. Davie, N. Edgardh & P. Pettersson, Ashgate, Farnham.

Ashencaen Crabtree, S., Hussain, F. & Spalek, B. (2008) *Islam and Social Work: Debating Values, Transforming Practice*, Policy Press, Bristol.

Australian Association of Social Workers (AASW) (1999) *Code of Ethics*, AASW, Canberra.

Australian Association of Social Workers (AASW) (2010) *Code of Ethics*, AASW, Canberra, [online]. Available at: http://www.aasw.asn.au/document/item/740, accessed 19 January 2011.

Barnett, C. K., Krell, T. C. & Sendry, J. (2000) 'Learning to learn about spirituality: a categorical approach to introducing the topic into management courses', *Journal of Management Education*, vol. 24, pp. 562–579.

Bowpitt, G. (1998) 'Evangelical Christianity, secular humanism and the genesis of British social work', *British Journal of Social Work*, vol. 28, pp. 675–693.

Bowpitt, G. (2000) 'Working with creative creatures: towards a Christian paradigm for social work theory with some practical implications', *British Journal of Social Work*, vol. 30, pp. 349–364.

Breward, I. (1988) *Australia: 'The Most Godless Place Under Heaven?'*, Beacon Hill Books, Melbourne.

Camilleri, P. & Winkworth, G. (2004) 'Mapping the Catholic social services', *Australasian Catholic Record*, vol. 81, pp. 184–197.

Canda, E. R. & Furman, D. L. (1999) *Spiritual Diversity in Social Work Practice: The Heart of Helping*, The Free Press, New York.

Clark, J. L. (2006) 'Listening for meaning: a research-based model for attending to spirituality, culture and worldview in social work practice', *Critical Social Work*, vol. 7, no. 1.

Crisp, B. R. (2009) 'Beyond the seminary: new frontiers for teaching spirituality', *Religious Education*, vol. 104, pp. 4–17.

Crisp, B. R. (2010a) *Spirituality and Social Work*, Ashgate, Farnham.

Crisp, B. R. (2010b) 'Catholic agencies: making a distinct contribution to Australian social welfare provision?', *Australasian Catholic Record*, vol. 87, pp. 440–451.

Dezerotes, D. S. (2006) 'Spirituality and religiosity: neglected factors in social work practice', *Arete*, vol. 20, pp. 1–15.

Doel, M., Allmark, P., Conway, P., Cowburn, M., Flynn, M., Nelson, P. & Tod, A. (2009) *Professional Boundaries: Research Report*, Centre for Health and Social Care Research, Sheffield Hallam University, Sheffield.

Edgardh, N. & Pettersson, P. (2010) 'The Church of Sweden: a church for all, especially the most vulnerable', in *Welfare and Religion in 21st Century Europe: Volume 1 Configuring the Connections*, eds A. Bäckström, G. Davie, N. Edgardh & P. Pettersson, Ashgate, Farnham.

Ferris, E. (2005) 'Faith-based and secular humanitarian organizations', *International Review of the Red Cross*, vol. 87, pp. 311–325.

Furman, L. D., Benson, P. W., Canda, E. R. & Grimwood, C. (2005) 'A comparative international analysis of religion and spirituality in social work: a survey of UK and US social workers', *Social Work Education*, vol. 24, pp. 813–839.

Furness, S. & Gilligan, P. (2010) *Religion, Belief and Social Work: Making a Difference*, Policy Press, Bristol.

Gale, F., Bolzan, N. & McRae-McMahon, D. (eds) (2007) *Spirited Practices: Spirituality and the Helping Professions*, Allen and Unwin, Crows Nest, NSW.

Gardner, F. (2006) *Working with Human Service Organisations: Creating Connections for Practice*, Oxford University Press, South Melbourne.

Gilbert, P. (2007) 'Engaging hearts and minds … and the spirit', *Journal of Integrated Care*, vol. 15, no. 4, pp. 20–25.

Gilligan, P. (2003) '"It isn't discussed". Religion, belief and practice teaching: missing components of cultural competence in social work', *Journal of Practice Teaching*, vol. 5, pp. 75–95.

Gollnick, J. (2005) *Religion and Spirituality in the Life Cycle*, Peter Lang, New York.

Goździak, E. M. (2002) 'Spiritual emergency room: the role of religion and spirituality in the resettlement of Kosovar Albanians', *Journal of Refugee Studies*, vol. 15, pp. 136–152.

Graham, J. R. (2007) 'The Haven, 1878–1939: a Toronto charity's transition from a religious to a professional social work ethos', in *Spirituality and Social Work: Selected Canadian Readings*, eds J. Coates, J. R. Graham, B. Swartzentruber & B. Ouellette, Canadian Scholars Press, Toronto.

Hafford-Letchfield, T. (2009) *Management and Organisations in Social Work*. 2nd edn. Learning Matters, Exeter.

Hay, D. & Nye, R. (2006) *The Spirit of the Child*. revised edn. Jessica Kingsley Publishers, London.

Hodge, D. R. (2002) 'Does social work oppress evangelical Christians? A "new class" analysis of society and social work', *Social Work*, vol. 47, pp. 401–414.

Hodge, D. R. (2005) 'Spirituality in social work education: a development and discussion of goals that flow from the profession's ethical mandates', *Social Work Education*, vol. 24, pp. 37–55.

Hodge, D. R. (2007) 'Advocating for persecuted people of faith: a social justice imperative', *Families in Society*, vol. 88, pp. 255–262.

Holloway, M. & Moss, B. (2010) *Spirituality and Social Work*, Palgrave Macmillan, Basingstoke.

International Association of Schools of Social Work (IASSW) & International Federation of Social Work (IFSW) (2004) *Global Standards for the Education and Training of the Social Work Profession* [online]. Available at: http://www.ifsw.org/cm_data/GlobalSocialWorkStandards2005.pdf, accessed 6 August 2010.

Lee, B. Y. & Newberg, A. B. (2005) 'Religion and health: a review and critical analysis', *Zygon*, vol. 40, pp. 443–468.

Lindsay, R. (2002) *Recognizing Spirituality: The Interface between Faith and Social Work*, University of Western Australia Press, Crawley.

Mathews, I. (2009) *Social Work and Spirituality*, Learning Matters, Exeter.

Melville, R. & McDonald, C. (2006) 'Faith-based organisations and contemporary welfare', *Australian Journal of Social Issues*, vol. 41, pp. 69–85.

Moss, B. (2002) 'Spirituality: a personal perspective', in *Loss and Grief: A Guide for Human Services Practitioners*, ed. N. Thompson, Palgrave, Basingstoke.

Moss, B. (2005) 'Thinking outside the box: religion and spirituality in social work education and practice', *Implicit Religion*, vol. 8, pp. 40–52.

Nash, M. & Stewart, B. (eds) (2002) *Spirituality and Social Care: Contributing to Personal and Community Well-being*, Jessica Kingsley Publishers, London.

Pessi, A. B. (2010) 'The church as a place of encounter: communality and the good life in Finland', in *Welfare and Religion in 21st Century Europe: Volume 1 Configuring the Connections*, eds A. Bäckström, G. Davie, N. Edgardh & P. Pettersson, Ashgate, Farnham.

Rizer, J. M. & McColley, K. J. (1996) 'Attitudes and practices regarding spirituality and religion held by graduate social work students', *Social Work and Christianity*, vol. 23, pp. 53–65.

Salvation Army (2010) *Fact and Fiction about Salvation Army History* [online]. Available at: http://www.salvationarmy.org.au/about-us_65047/history-and-heritage/fact-and-fiction-.html, accessed 28 May 2010.

Sheridan, M. J., Bullis, R. K., Adcock, C. R., Berlin, S. D. & Miller, P. C. (1992) 'Practitioners' personal and professional attitudes and behavior toward religion and spirituality: issues for education and practice', *Journal of Social Work Education*, vol. 28, pp. 190–203.

Sheridan, M. J., Wilmer, C. M. & Atcheson, L. (1994) 'Inclusion of religion and spirituality in the social work curriculum: a study of faculty views', *Journal of Social Work Education*, vol. 30, pp. 363–376.

Swinton, J. (2001) *Spirituality and Mental Health Care: Rediscovering a 'Forgotten' Dimension*, Jessica Kingsley Publishers, London.

Tacey, D. (2003) *The Spirituality Revolution: The Emergence of Contemporary Spirituality*, HarperCollins Publishers, Sydney.

Tangenberg, K. M. (2005) 'Faith-based human services initiatives: considerations for social work theory and practice', *Social Work*, vol. 50, pp. 197–206.

Valasik, C. (2010) 'Church–state relations in France in the field of welfare: a hidden complementarity', in *Welfare and Religion in 21st Century Europe: Volume 1 Configuring the Connections*, eds A. Bäckström, G. Davie, N. Edgardh & P. Pettersson, Ashgate, Farnham.

Vanderwoerd, J. R. (2006) 'Threat from the south: is American religion bad news for Canadian social welfare?', *Critical Social Work*, vol. 7, no. 1.

Wagler-Martin, W. (2005) 'Listening to our stillness: giving our voice to our spirituality (spirituality and clinical practice)', *Critical Social Work*, vol. 6, no. 2.

Winkworth, G. & Camilleri, P. (2004) 'Keeping the faith: the impact of human services restructuring on Catholic social welfare services', *Australian Journal of Social Issues*, vol. 39, pp. 315–328.

Work–Life Balance: Practitioner Well-Being in the Social Work Education Curriculum

Christa Fouché & Kathy Martindale

Drawing on the debates of 'work–life balance' (WLB), subjective well-being (SWB) and life satisfaction (LS), this article seeks to reflect on the issue of social work practitioner well-being in the social work education curriculum. The authors argue that, to enable the elusive 'work–life balance' for social work practitioners, we need conversations about the life domains that define balance for each individual. Discussions about life satisfaction or dissatisfaction in social work education can be a crucial starting point for ongoing assessment of aspects of balance for the individual as part of the future workforce. We propose that awareness of, and dialogue about, core domains of life satisfaction during training will also eventually enable more effective management of stress and burnout and quality of service delivery in practice, as well as provide a framework for professional development and career progression of practitioners.

We adopt a three-fold discussion: first, we explore the meaning of work–life balance and sketch the implications thereof within social work; second, we trace the relationship between work–life balance, subjective well-being and life satisfaction; and finally, we outline issues for social work education and suggest practices that can enhance practitioner well-being in the longer term and promote safe habits within social work education.

Introduction

It is widely recognised that practitioners in the caring professions, in the nature of the jobs' demands, deal with a range of stressful experiences on a daily basis. It is increasingly clear though, that issues rooted in various aspects of the organisation and in the context of service delivery are the real stressors that impact on job satisfaction, professional commitment and retention. These stressors include staff shortages and demanding workloads; excessive paperwork and administrative burdens; limited resources and inadequate training, more so than critical incident stressors and stressors related to vicarious trauma (Regehr *et al.*, 2000; Thompson, 2004). Collings and Murray (1996) report pressure involved in planning and reaching work targets as the most powerful predictor of stress for social workers. Highly relevant to the experiences of social work practitioners, Goh and Watt (2003) report the main stressors experienced by nurses transitioning from 'dependent on' at university to 'depended on' in practice, as managing multiple roles and personal stressors alongside the unrealistic expectations of colleagues.

The management of stress and burnout, staff retention, practice conduct, productivity and quality of service delivery are known challenges for managers in the social services. A range of measures are promoted to manage stressors or their negative effects, including induction, supervision, workload management, continuing professional development, managerial practices of recognition and collegiality and reflective practice or improved practice of self-awareness (IFSW, 2010). The impact of effective supervision in fostering beneficial and in limiting detrimental outcomes for workers is particularly well documented and promoted (Mor Barak *et al.*, 2009). Giffords (2009) suggests that social work managers ought to develop a greater understanding of organisational and professional commitment because of its link to organisational effectiveness amongst other things. Simultaneously, discussions about the cost of unhealthy workplaces (incorporating both physical and psychological health) are increasingly balanced with discussions about the benefits of positive practice environments (WHPA, 2008). Shier and Graham (2011) claim that subjective well-being can be a key resource in helping social workers practise more effectively. It is within this context that the notion of the balance between work and life has become a source of much discussion. The notion of work–life balance is sometimes viewed as a stressor (by lack thereof) and sometimes offered as a strategy (through policies enabling it).

Work–life balance has received growing attention professionally and commercially across a number of fields over the last decade. Supporting the development of work–life balance raises a series of interrelated questions: what is work and how does that differ from life?; can the perfect balance between work and life outside of work be achieved?; how is work best shaped to allow balance?; and how can employers fulfil their obligation to ensure work entertains the notion of a balance with other life commitments? These are not simply instrumental questions but rather inherently philosophical issues that lie beyond typical discussions about how work–life balance can be achieved. This article is not aimed at addressing these issues, but points towards the value of conversations about practitioner well-being in the social work education curriculum by: exploring the meaning of work–life balance (and the implications thereof) within social work; making transparent the relationship between work–life balance, subjective well-being and life satisfaction; and discussing implications for thinking about these positive psychology practices in the development of social work practitioner well-being. We highlight issues for social work education and suggest practices that can enhance practitioner well-being and promote safe habits.

Work–Life Balance Defined

An Internet search for the construct 'work–life balance' can produce easily in excess of 40 million results, which is a clear indication that this is not only a scholarly construct, but also a very popular and well-supported commercial concept. Judging from these websites, many individuals, organisations and even governments are supportive of the concept and it is widely presented and discussed as a solution to issues faced by many in the paid workforce. It is also regarded as a valuable form of workplace organisation that employers should recognise and support. Work–life balance initiatives are seen as 'having the potential to be a win–win for both individuals and organizations' (Barnett and Hall, 2001, p. 192), in that through the implementation of work–life balance policies, organisations can ensure that employees deliver the best possible input while also meeting family, work and community responsibilities.

However, some authors do offer a critical view of the concept. Dupuis (2007) demonstrates numerous problems associated with the term, stating that the concept sets up a false binary between 'work' on the one hand and 'life' on the other. She continues to argue that the concept is not applicable to all workers, and is, in fact, irrelevant to some. In unpacking the three parts to this construct (work, life and balance) linguistically, this binary becomes very clear. 'Work' is popularly regarded as labour or employment and associated with an economically active population: '...the supply of labour for the production of economic goods and services ...' (International Labour Organisation, 2005). A distinction can broadly be made between standard work and non-standard work, where standard work has been defined as paid employment delivered at the employer's workplace with a direct relationship between employer and employee and non-standard work defined as a variation from 'standard work' through varying hours of work, tenure of employment, employee/employer relationships and the location of the work (Dupuis, 2007). The dictionary meaning of 'life', expectedly, indicates the course of existence of an individual; the condition of living or the state of being alive; the period between birth and the present time. It is also broadly defined as a characteristic state or mode of living; 'social life'; 'city life'; 'political life'; 'work life' (http://www.dictionary.net/life). Therefore definitions about life often include reference to life domains and, increasingly, reference to domains of life satisfaction or quality of life (Cummins, 2003), as will be discussed in more detail below. 'Balance' is seen as finding a state of equilibrium; an intermediate position or compromise; or the action to weigh alternatives perceived and communicated as the 'ideal state' (http://www.dictionary.net/balance).

The concept 'work–life balance' is promoted as a practice valued by employees and that employers should recognise in workplace policies and practices aimed at promoting a better balance between paid work and life outside of work (Department of Labour,

2004). In the paid workforce, work–life balance thus predominantly means having sufficient time for family and other 'life' obligations. As Dupuis (2007) states, the common image conjured up by the word 'balance' is one of scales, in which weights on one side match equally with a commodity being weighed on the other. When the weights on the one side correspond to the weight of the commodity on the other, a balance has been achieved. Taking this view of balance one might therefore expect the term work–life balance to mean an equal balance between 'work' on the one hand and 'life' on the other.

Looking critically at the concept in this way it does raise a number of questions pertinent to social work. Are the concepts of 'work' and 'worker' restricted to paid employment? Is work–life balance therefore irrelevant for people in 'unpaid' work? As some categories of work are excluded or marginal to the definition of 'economic activity' (such as domestic work or voluntary work), do these then become irrelevant to the debates around work–life balance? And most importantly, how do we consider work–life balance when life becomes work (as in the case of providing fulltime care for a relative) (Waring and Fouché, 2007)? This creates the context for discussions about the notion of work–life balance and related concepts as a measure for managing stressors, promoting safe habits and as a key resource to help social workers practise more effectively. We will now turn to a discussion of the relationship between work–life balance, subjective well-being and life satisfaction.

Subjective Well-Being and Life Satisfaction

The study of subjective well-being is embedded in the new field of investigation known as Positive Psychology (Seligman and Csikszentmihalyi, 2000). Positive Psychology focuses on the positive end of psychological well-being and provides a counterbalance to the negative affect and 'pathology' dominance found in psychology until the mid-1970s (Frisch, 2000). The Positive Psychology approach is concerned with the study and investigation of what makes experiences of life pleasant and, thus, looks at issues such as pleasure, interest, joy, happiness and of satisfaction in a range of circumstances ranging from the biological level of the individual through to the societal level (Kahneman et al., 1999).

Subjective well-being is globally the term most used to describe how people generally feel about their life. It captures the experiences of a person's life that are important to them, rather than the indirect measure of satisfaction that objective social indicators provide (e.g. Gross National Product or income levels, access to health services, crime rates ...), or the judgment of experts. Throughout the social sciences field subjective well-being has gained considerable importance and has become a major research interest. This interest is also reflected in the general population, as demonstrated in a study of college students across 17 countries by Diener (2000). In this study students not only reported that happiness and life satisfaction were very important (more so than money) but that they also frequently thought about these two constructs. Increasingly the debates in this field seem to have particular relevance for dialogue about work–life balance and, as argued in this article, for social work students in their consideration of wellness.

As visually presented in Figure 1, subjective well-being consists of four interrelated components: life satisfaction, domain satisfaction, pleasant affect and unpleasant affect (Diener and Lucas, 1999). Thus, subjective well-being is the assessment of either cognitive judgments of life satisfaction or affective evaluations of moods and emotions, or a combination of both, that individuals make about their lives. Life satisfaction, pleasant affect and unpleasant affect are related but are also conceptually separate and need to be studied independently for a complete overall picture of subjective well-being. Consistent with this view, Diener *et al.* (1999, p. 277) defined subjective well-being as 'a general area of scientific interest rather than a single specific construct'. They argued that, as a general construct, subjective well-being could be divided into a number of components, such as satisfaction with one's current life, with past life and with future expected life or with satisfaction with specific domains of life (e.g. marriage, work, recreation or friendship). Similarly, pleasant affect can be divided into specific emotions, such as joy, happiness, and affection, while unpleasant affect can be divided into specific negative emotions such as guilt, sadness and anger (Diener *et al.*, 1999).

Subjective well-being can be assessed at a global level, with a single question: 'How satisfied are you with your life-as-a-whole?' (Andrews and Withey, 1976), and more explicitly by asking satisfaction questions about various life domains (e.g. marital satisfaction, work satisfaction), which provides unique information regarding an individual's overall well-being. This, then, links closely with the notion of work–life balance, with the understanding that one would aim to balance satisfaction in the work domain with satisfaction in other domains of life—whatever those domains may be for any given individual. As such, life satisfaction becomes an important component of subjective well-being. The cognitive component of subjective well-being is conceptualised as life satisfaction (Andrews and Withey, 1976). Life satisfaction is defined by Pavot *et al.* (1991) as 'a global evaluation by the person on his or her life' (p. 150). As a global measure life satisfaction has been found to be both reliable (Larsen *et al.*, 1985) and consistent when measured in Western countries (Cummins, 1995, 2003). Life satisfaction is viewed as a conscious process in which an individual makes judgments about their life quality based on their own unique set of criteria and

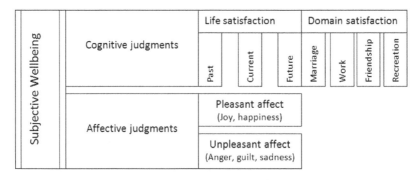

Figure 1   The Interrelated Components of Subjective Well-Being.

experiences (Larsen *et al.*, 1985). That is, an individual has a particular standard that they perceive as appropriate to them and when making life satisfaction judgments they compare the circumstances of their life to that standard. The degree to which life conditions match their own unique set of standards, the greater the level of life satisfaction experienced. Thus, life satisfaction is a subjective judgment, rather than a judgment based on externally imposed or objective standards.

The congruence between an individual's perceived satisfaction and their life circumstances has generally been described using discrepancy theory, the most comprehensive discrepancy model of which was proposed by Michalos (1985) in his Multiple Discrepancy Theory (MDT). This theory proposes that satisfaction is a function of the discrepancy between seven comparisons. These are the perceived difference between what one has versus:

- what one wants;
- what others have;
- the best one has had in the past;
- what one expected to have in the past;
- what one expects to have in the future;
- what one deserves; and
- what one needs.

Individual differences of personality and life experiences produce different desired circumstances and self-standards and thus discrepancies between these aspects will differ greatly from one individual to another. There are many psychological well-being scales associated with these complex and interrelated constructs (Diener *et al.*, 2010). In discussing life satisfaction, Lucas *et al.* (1996) argue that, while the concept of life satisfaction is theoretically different from the amount of positive or negative affect a person experiences, the constructs affect and life satisfaction are interrelated in that, during the process of making life satisfaction judgments, individuals tend to rely on their mood as an indicator of overall satisfaction (Schwartz and Strack, 1991). Life satisfaction (happiness) is highly correlated to social competence, social skills, connectedness, social relationships with others and participation in work and leisure activities (Schalock and Felce, 2004).

As noted by Diener (2000), happy people, on average, appear to be more productive and sociable. Clearly, high levels of subjective well-being may well be highly beneficial for a society and therefore a valued goal for which to strive. This is true not only for clients and communities, but also for the practitioners doing the work. The importance of subjective well-being to optimal human functioning is described by Headey and Wearing (1992) as being a fundamental objective of life in which people exhibit a strong desire to both attain and experience high levels of well-being. We argue that this is also an important aim for social work practitioners and, as mentioned earlier, a measure for managing stressors, promoting safe habits and a key resource to help social workers assess work–life balance. We now turn to the relevance of this in social work education.

Conversations on Work, Life and Balance in the Context of Practitioner Education

As has been demonstrated in the discussions above, the notion of finding a balance between work and life for social work practitioners becomes linked to a need for conversations about the life domains that define balance for each individual. As individual differences of personality and life experiences produce different desired circumstances and self-standards, there can be no one solution for finding a work–life balance. On the contrary, one might expect the term work–life balance not to mean an equal balance between 'work' on the one hand and 'life' on the other, but a balance of important life domains. As such, discussions about life satisfaction or dissatisfaction during social work training can be a crucial starting point for ongoing assessment of aspects of balance for the individual as part of the future workforce and to promote safe habits during education.

Discussions of life domains and life satisfaction are not at all unfamiliar in social work education, as personal knowledge incorporating values, culture, gender, education and the importance of family, relationships and spirituality is often promoted in the curriculum (Maidment and Egan, 2004; Trevithick, 2008; Connolly and Harms, 2009; Beddoe and Maidment, 2009). However, there is relatively little reference to this as part of practitioner well-being and limited reference to specific practices to enhance practitioner well-being in the social work education curriculum. In reflecting on the findings of a study in the use of mindfulness as a tool, Shier and Graham (2011) state that the act of being mindful about identity, capabilities and environments might usefully predict higher levels of overall subjective well-being for practising social workers. Yager and Tovar-Blank (2007) warn, however, that some educators may develop crucial self-awareness and the use of self as a therapeutic tool, but even these directions of training can be considered without a conscious effort to consider the overall wellness of the student. Similarly, there is an abundance of material on stress management and self-care strategies in the caring professions (Collins, 2008; Christopher and Maris, 2010) and particularly in child protection or statutory services (Regehr *et al.*, 2000), but most of these pertain to practitioners in the workforce and although some highlight professional and personal well-being in the education of practitioners, promoting safe habits around well-being is hardly ever the focus (Moran and Hughes, 2006; Yager and Tovar-Blank, 2007).

The importance of reflections on life domains and life satisfaction in managing practitioner well-being should be incorporated within the social work education curriculum where content about personal knowledge, values, culture, gender, relationships, spirituality and the importance of reflection and self-care are addressed. This can feasibly be done in several places, including units on lifespan and human development, social work theory, professional development and supervision or within the context of organisational management. However, the most important place would certainly be in social work field education curricula where the opportunity exists to actively engage with students about their own potential vulnerabilities in this regard.

One focus of subjective well-being research has been to unravel the uncertainty about which variables cause subjective well-being and which variables are consequences. Some of the variables that have been proposed as causes of subjective well-being are domain satisfaction, social support, major life events and referenced standards (e.g. expectations, aspirations, and sense of equity) (Headey *et al.*, 1991). Examination of life domains highlights specific areas of vulnerability for imbalance and provides direction for possible intervention in order to enhance a person's quality of life or to attain balance. This means that specific domains can be used as diagnostic indicators, as a low mean score in particular domains can indicate a potential vulnerability for disrupted balance. Such indicated areas can then be targeted for intervention and practices that can enhance practitioner well-being in the longer term can be instituted. Preparing students for, and supporting them on, field placements certainly seems an appropriate time to engage in these discussions.

It is important to note though, that we are not arguing for addressing and improving the wellness of students. In fact, according to Myers *et al.*, (2003), one can expect that senior counselling students (and this will be true for many students in social work and other caring professions) may well experience greater wellness than the general population. We argue for the inclusion of content about subjective well-being in the social work education curriculum that will enable awareness of, and dialogue about, core domains of life satisfaction in order to promote safe habits and for this to preferably happen within the field education curriculum. This will not only allow an individual practitioner, or practitioner-to-be, to consider their own life domains and the importance of each, but will eventually enable them to articulate these appropriately to the extent that supervisors and managers will have a clear view of the importance of some life domains when weighted against others. This will enable supervisors and managers to more effectively manage stressors and burnout by addressing the domains that matter most. In doing so, one can assume that more effective and safe practice may result.

We have mentioned earlier that subjective well-being can be assessed with the single question: 'How satisfied are you with your life-as-a-whole?' (Andrews and Withey, 1976) and also more explicitly by asking satisfaction questions about various life domains (e.g. marital satisfaction, work satisfaction). Introducing content on life domains to the social work curriculum as appropriate and then expecting students to explore the question, 'How satisfied are you with your life-as-a-whole?' in a reflective journal, will assist them to grasp the value of assessment of their life domains and the ongoing balancing thereof when they join the workforce. Yager and Tovar-Blank (2007) suggest that, in promoting student wellness during training, educators should clearly communicate that perfection is not the goal of wellness. Enriching discussions about domain satisfaction with a dialogue on past, current and future experiences of life satisfaction may enable cognitive judgments about subjective well-being that recognise the life domains that contribute to one's subjective well-being rather than just 'achieving a balance' of work and life outside of work.

Conclusion

We have explored the binary meaning of the work–life balance and the implications thereof within social work, and we have traced the relationship between work–life

127

balance, subjective well-being and life satisfaction. From this, the importance of subjective well-being to optimal human functioning became clear and we argued that this is also an important aim for social work practitioners. Within this context, we posed that an appropriate time to explore the aim and measures to achieve it will be during education, and in particular, in the field education curriculum. Not only are these issues crucial to beginning practice and the transition of students to professional practice, but they are important for practitioners in managing their organisational environments and self-managing their identity and expertise. If we agree that consideration of work–life balance is a mechanism to counter stress, fatigue and burnout as constant threats, we need to value conversations on the life domains that define 'balance' for each individual.

Subjective well-being levels can be defeated by negative 'life events', particularly when these events occur in domains of our life that are significantly important to us, such as work or family life. This has huge implications for social work in as far as an individual's satisfaction with domains outside of work will impact on their satisfaction with life (including their work life), while their satisfaction with work will impact on satisfaction with life. Yager and Tovar-Blank (2007) remind us that an imbalance between the personal, social, physical, spiritual, and occupational domains of our lives is inevitable, but as social workers we can successfully address moment-to-moment adjustments approximating a wellness-focused balance. Allowing these conversations in the social work education curriculum may be one more way to promote safe habits and eventually enhance practitioner well-being in practice.

References

Andrews, F. M. & Withey, S. B. (1976) *Social Indicators of Well-Being: Americans' Perception of Life Quality*, Plenum Press, New York.

Barnett, R. & Hall, T. (2001) 'How to use reduced hours to win the war for talent', *Organizational Dynamics*, vol. 29, no. 3, pp. 192–210.

Beddoe, L. & Maidment, J. (2009) *Mapping Knowledge for Social Work Practice*, Cengage Learning, South Melbourne.

Christopher, J. C. & Maris, J. A. (2010) 'Integrating mindfulness as self-care into counselling and psychotherapy training', *Counselling and Psychotherapy Research*, vol. 10, no. 2, pp. 114–125.

Collings, J. A. & Murray, P. J. (1996) 'Predictors of stress amongst social workers: an empirical study', *British Journal of Social Work*, vol. 26, pp. 375–387.

Collins, S. (2008) 'Statutory social workers: stress, job satisfaction, coping, social support and individual differences', *British Journal of Social Work*, vol. 38, no. 6, pp. 1173–1193.

Connolly, M. & Harms, L. (eds) (2009) *Social Work: Contexts and Practice*, 2nd edn. Oxford University Press, London.

Cummins, R. A. (1995) 'On the trail of the gold standard for subjective well-being', *Social Indicators Research*, vol. 35, pp. 179–200.

Cummins, R. A. (2003) 'Normative life satisfaction: measurement issues and a homeostatic model', *Social Indicators Research*, vol. 64, no. 2, pp. 225–256.

Department of Labour (2004) *Achieving Balanced Lives and Employment: What New Zealanders are Saying about Work–Life Balance* [online]. Available at: http://www.dol.govt.nz/PDFs/wlb-consultation-summary.pdf, accessed 29 October 2010.

Diener, E. (2000) 'Subjective well-being: the science of happiness and a proposal for a national index', *American Psychologist*, vol. 55, no. 1, pp. 34–43.

Diener, E. & Lucas, R. E. (1999) 'Personality and subjective well-being', in *Well-Being: The Foundations of Hedonic Psychology*, eds D. Kahneman, E. Diener & N. Schwarz, Russell Sage Foundations, New York, pp. 213–229.

Diener, E., Suh, E. M., Lucas, R. E. & Smith, H. L. (1999) 'Subjective well-being: three decades of progress', *Psychological Bulletin*, vol. 125, no. 2, pp. 276–302.

Diener, E., Wirtz, D., Tov, W., Kim-Prieto, C., Choi, D., Oishi, S. & Biswas-Diener, R. (2010) 'New well-being measures: short scales to assess flourishing and positive and negative feelings', *Social Indicators Research*, vol. 97, no. 2, pp. 143–156.

Dupuis, A. (2007) 'Work–life balance: rhetoric or "Reality"?', in *Managing Mayhem: Work Life Balance in New Zealand*, eds M. Waring & C. B. Fouche, Dunmore Press, Wellington.

Frisch, M. B. (2000) 'Improving mental and physical health care through quality of life therapy and assessment', in *Advances in Quality of Life Theory and Research*, Vol. 4, eds E. Diener & D. R. Rahtz, Kluwer Academic Publishers, Dordrecht, pp. 207–241.

Giffords, E. D. (2009) 'An examination of organizational commitment and professional commitment and the relationship to work environment, demographic and organizational factors', *Journal of Social Work*, vol. 9, no. 4, pp. 386–404.

Goh, K. & Watt, E. (2003) 'From "dependent on" to "depended on": the experience of transition from student to registered nurse in a private hospital graduate program', *Australian Journal of Advanced Nursing*, vol. 21, no. 1, pp. 14–20.

Headey, B., Veenhoven, R. & Wearing, A. (1991) 'Top-down versus bottom up theories of subjective well-being', *Social Indicators Research*, vol. 24, pp. 81–100.

Headey, B. & Wearing, A. (1992) *Understanding Happiness: A Theory of Subjective Wellbeing*, Longman Cheshire, Melbourne.

International Federation of Social Workers European Region E.V. (IFSW) (2010) *Standards in Social Work Practice Meeting Human Rights*, IFSW, Berlin.

International Labour Organisation (ILO) (2005) *ILO Thesaurus* [online]. Available at: http://www.ilo.org/public/libdoc/ILO-Thesaurus/english/tr2454.htm, accessed 29 October 2010.

Kahneman, D., Diener, E. & Schwarz, N. (eds) (1999) *Well-Being: The Foundations of Hedonic Psychology*, Russell Sage, New York.

Larsen, R. J., Diener, E. & Emmons, R. A. (1985) 'An evaluation of subjective well-being measures', *Social Indicators Research*, vol. 17, pp. 1–17.

Lucas, R. E., Diener, E. & Suh, E. (1996) 'Discriminant validity of well-being measures', *Journal of Personality and Social Psychology*, vol. 71, no. 3, pp. 616–628.

Maidment, J. & Egan, R. (eds) (2004) *Practice Skills in Social Work and Welfare: More Than Just Common Sense*, Allen & Unwin, Sydney.

Michalos, A. C. (1985) 'Multiple discrepancies theory (MDT)', *Social Indicators Research*, vol. 16, pp. 347–413.

Mor Barak, M. E., Travis, D. J., Pyun, H. & Xie, B. (2009) 'The impact of supervision on worker outcomes: a meta-analysis', *Social Service Review*, March, pp. 3–32 .

Moran, C. & Hughes, L. (2006) 'Coping with stress: social work students and humour', *Social Work Education*, vol. 25, no. 5, pp. 501–517.

Myers, J. E., Mobley, A. K. & Booth, C. S. (2003) 'Wellness of counseling students: practicing what we preach', *Counselor Education and Supervision*, vol. 42, no. 4, pp. 264–274.

Pavot, W., Diener, E., Colvin, C. R. & Sandvik, E. (1991) 'Further validation of the satisfaction with life scale: evidence for the cross-method convergence of well-being measures', *Journal of Personality Assessment*, vol. 57, no. 1, pp. 149–161.

Regehr, C., Leslie, B., Howe, P. & Chau, S. (2000) *Stressors in Child Welfare*, University of Toronto, Canada [online]. Available at: http://dev.cecw-cepb.ca/files/file/en/Stressors.pdf, accessed 29 October 2010.

Schalock, R. L. & Felce, D. (2004) 'Quality of life and subjective well-being: conceptual and measurement issues', in *International Handbook on Applied Research in Intellectual Disabilities*, eds E. Emerson, C. Hatton, T. Thompson & T. R. Parmenter, John Wiley & Sons, Chichester, West Sussex, pp. 261–279.

Schwartz, N. & Strack, F. (1991) 'Evaluating one's life: a judgement model of subjective well-being', in *Subjective Well-Being: An Interdisciplinary Perspective*, eds F. Strack, M. Argyle & N. Schwarz, Pergamon Press, Oxford, pp. 27–47.

Seligman, M. E. P. & Csikszentmihalyi, M. (2000) 'Positive psychology: an introduction', *American Psychologist*, vol. 55, no. 1, pp. 5–14.

Shier, M. L. & Graham, J. R. (2011) 'Mindfulness, subjective well-being, and social work: insight into their interconnection from social work practitioners', *Social Work Education*, vol. 30, no. 1, pp. 29–44.

Thompson, L. (2004) 'Burnout or secondary traumatic stress? The importance of self care for mental health professionals', *Irish Social Worker*, vol. 22, no. 1, pp. 15–16.

Trevithick, P. (2008) 'Revisiting the knowledge base of social work: a framework for practice', *British Journal of Social Work*, vol. 38, no. 6, pp. 1212–1237.

Waring, M. & Fouché, C. B. (eds) (2007) *Managing Mayhem: Work–Life Balance in New Zealand*, Dunmore Press, Wellington.

World Health Professional Alliance (WHPA) (2008) *Fact Sheet on Positive Practice Environments for Health Care Professionals* [online]. Available at: http://www.whpa.org/PPE_Fact_Health_Pro.pdf, accessed 29 October 2010.

Yager, G. G. & Tovar-Blank, Z. G. (2007) 'Wellness and counselor education', *Journal of Humanistic Counseling, Education & Development*, vol. 46, no. 2, pp. 142–153.

Do Challenges to Students' Beliefs, Values and Behaviour within Social Work Education Have an Impact on Their Sense of Well-Being?

Mel Hughes

This paper draws on the findings of a unitary appreciative inquiry which aimed to illuminate the unique experiences of five student social workers approaching qualification. It identifies the impact social work education had on their whole selves, their beliefs, values and behaviour, and the impact of this learning on their sense of well-being. The findings are summarised and presented within this paper as five individual profiles including the participants' own representations of this impact. The study found that their well-being was affected significantly by changes to their sense of self, changing relationships with others and heightened awareness of oppression and injustice. Whilst all reported positive outcomes resulting from personal, academic and professional achievement, all shared examples of where their learning had impacted negatively on relationships with friends and family. This had led to internal conflict as they sought to adjust to their new ways of thinking and the implications for their behaviour past and present. The participants believed that this was best supported within social work education when values and behaviours were modelled by staff, when educators acknowledged and understood the potential impact of learning and when networks for sharing experiences, seeking support and enabling slow, developmental change were available.

Introduction

This paper draws on the findings of a unitary appreciative inquiry (Cowling, 2001, 2004a, 2004b, 2005) which aimed to illuminate the unique experiences of the student social work participants, in relation to the impact that they believe social work education has had on their whole selves, their beliefs, values and behaviour, and the impact of this learning on themselves. It represents as close a picture as possible of their experiences and the implications of their experience for social work education. The research is based on a holistic view of learners that recognises that their identity goes beyond that of student or social worker. It acknowledges the multiple aspects of their 'whole selves' such as physical, spiritual and emotional, and of the interconnectedness between them and their environment. It recognises that challenges and changes to their beliefs, values and behaviour during their education may have a significant impact on their whole selves and their lives. The research study is underpinned by educational theory developed by Rogers (1969), Knowles (1984) and Mezirow (1996) amongst others as they recognise the proactive, individualised processes of learning where knowledge is internalised and made sense of through the lens of our previous experiences. As such, learning is likely to affect all aspects of our lives as our knowledge and outlook on life changes. Whilst the research study focussed on the broader question of what impact this learning had on their lives, a range of evidence emerged regarding the impact of their learning on their sense of well-being. The insight, learning, knowledge and practice development gained by recognising and appreciating their perceptions is explored within the wider context of social work education. Options for acknowledging and supporting students through this transition are discussed.

Background

As a lecturer on an undergraduate social work programme, I wanted to explore whether the focus within social work education on values, beliefs and behaviour, and the need to align these with the values of the profession, has an impact on the person outside of the classroom. Gardner (2001, p. 29) for example comments that 'if people start to change their views about gender issues in class, this is likely to affect how they see gender issues at home so affect significant relationships'. My professional values as a social work practitioner are to recognise the person within the context of their lives; to seek an understanding of their experiences from the person themselves; and to negotiate with them, as much as possible, regarding the most appropriate way to intervene. As this approach is based on respect and on viewing individuals as unique and their own best expert, I have sought to transfer this approach and value base to my role as educator when working with students. The study illuminates these experiences by focussing on students completing their undergraduate social work education. The students shared a number of experiences which can increase our insight into the impact of their learning experience on their sense of well-being.

Well-Being

Well-being as identified within this study relates to a student's sense of well-being and as such includes the different aspects of physical, mental and social well-being referred to by the Ottawa Charter for health promotion (WHO, 1986). The study did not seek to differentiate between these as it took a holistic approach which seeks to view the person as a whole and not as reducible parts. This is congruent with the approach the study used of unitary appreciative inquiry which seeks to gain the 'deepest possible understanding of (an experience) and its relationship to the person's life' (Cowling, 2004b, p. 289). The Ottawa Charter states that 'to reach a state of complete physical, mental and social well-being, an individual or group must be able to identify and realize aspirations, to satisfy needs, and to change and cope with their environment'. The participants in the study expressed an overwhelmingly positive outcome to their education and the impact on their sense of well-being in terms of meeting aspirations and satisfying need but expressed difficult experiences during the process of adapting to their environment and to the changes in self.

Context

Social work education, as with other professional education, is not restricted to the passive acquisition of knowledge but must also focus on the personal and professional development of skills and values and the application of that learning to the person's practice. The aim of social work education is to improve the quality of the workforce through the development of competent, confident, self-aware and reflective practitioners who are able to cope with the pressures, demands and risks of the work whilst maintaining a professional value base which places service users and carers at the heart of the process.

To achieve this, contemporary social work education and social work practice is guided in England by recommendations by Lord Laming (2003, 2009), The Social Work Taskforce (2009) and the *National Occupational Standards for Social Work* (TOPSS, 2002). These place an increased emphasis on the individual, on personal qualities, on the need to critically reflect, and on the increasing use of self. As Cournoyer (2000, p. 35) states 'social work practice involves the conscious and deliberate use of oneself; you become the medium through which knowledge, attitudes and skills are conveyed' (cited in Reupert, 2007, p. 107). The Social Work Taskforce makes recommendations for entry into the profession which emphasise the need for social work students to have particular personal qualities such as 'insight, common sense, confidence, resilience, empathy and the use of authority' (2009, p. 17). Service users and carers have emphasised the need for social workers to possess personal qualities such as warmth, empathy, understanding, and for them to be punctual, reliable and trustworthy (Skills for Care, 2002). The *National Occupational Standards* for social workers in England include a number of value requirements such as the need for social workers to have an 'awareness of own values, prejudices, ethical dilemmas, conflict of interests and implications for practice' (TOPSS, 2002, p. 63).

Whilst some emphasis has been placed on recruiting students who already possess these qualities and values, the role for social work education is to assess individual students' values, beliefs and behaviours and to enable them to align these with those of the profession or prevent them from qualifying if they do not. This brings into scrutiny personal aspects of a person's sense of self and identity which will inevitably have an impact on their whole selves and potentially on their sense of well-being.

There is evidence to demonstrate that significant changes do take place as students experience a range of catalysts which lead to shifts in their beliefs, values and frames of reference (Argyris and Schon, 1974; Mezirow, 1996; Johns, 2005). There has been a significant increase in the range of social work literature relating to teaching and enabling the development of skills in critical reflection (Fook, 2004; Gould and Baldwin, 2004; White *et al.*, 2006 amongst others) which can help students to make sense of these shifts and changes. Exploration into the impact of these changes, transformations and consolidations on the person themselves, however, remains minimal. For those participating in this study, the shifts in values were perceived as having a significant and, at times, life-changing impact. The transformative nature of social work education is touched on by Collins *et al.* (2010) when identifying causes of stress amongst social work students but other than this study, it seems that the literature is limited to research which has focussed only on aspects of a person's life, such as reasons for retention (Hafford-Letchfield, 2007), parenting (Green-Lister, 2003) and spiritual well-being (Kamya, 2000). There has been little focus on the whole person within the context of their lives and the impact that changes to values, beliefs and behaviour may have on their sense of well-being.

Perhaps nearer to the mark is the literature relating to social work education and personal growth as this recognises changes to the person themselves. Pardeck and McCallister (1991, p. 383) identified that 'personal growth and development as well as intellectual growth of students are major goals of social work education', however their assessment in the early 1990s, of student's personal growth through completion of self-expression, generalised contentment and self-esteem scales, suggested that undergraduate social work education had 'little or no effect on the personal growth or development of students' (p. 385). They compare this to a study by Cournoyer in 1983 where social work students were assessed as having a decrease in assertiveness after their social work training (as a result of what Cournoyer termed 'battered student syndrome'). More recent studies such as Collins *et al.* (2010) report a high level of students feeling they were a 'person of worth' and yet over a quarter of the students in their study reported negative attitudes about themselves such as feeling dissatisfied with themselves, not feeling proud of the people they were and not feeling that they were as good as other people. This poses the question of whether we are losing sight of the person (the student), their perceptions, needs and well-being within this process. Seeking to recognise and understand the impact that the process of learning and transition has on the whole person by illuminating their experience has the potential to improve both the experience for students and the outcomes for the profession.

Methodology

The study used a unitary appreciative inquiry (UAI) to gain these insights and perspectives. UAI is a relatively new qualitative approach still being developed by W. Richard Cowling originally for use within mental health nursing research and practice. Cowling argues that by understanding and appreciating life patterns, wholeness and uniqueness, practitioners can seek to improve 'the lives of individuals, families, groups and communities' (2005, p. 94). Whilst it seeks patterns which reflect the wholeness, essence and uniqueness of a particular individual or group, reflection on these representations and patterns 'can provide a way of understanding human life, conditions and situations' (Cowling, 2001, p. 35). As such they can be used to inform our understanding of the particular context as well as the particular person. UAI seeks to achieve this understanding by generating and collecting a range of data regarding the person or group's experience; representations of that experience using methods of creative expression, e.g. music, art, storytelling; and the participants' views on the implications of that knowledge for themselves and others. It creates a synopsis of these data in the form of an appreciative profile which can then be used for further reflection and analysis by participants, the researcher and others.

Method

The five participants were self-selecting from the final year cohort of the undergraduate social work degree for which I am lecturer. As the participants were known to me, a number of factors relating to insider research (Mercer, 2007; Coghlan, 2007; Gunasekara, 2007; Darra, 2008) and informed consent (Miller and Crabtree, 1999; Malone, 2003) were considered when seeking ethical approval and these were shared with potential participants prior to volunteering. Participants had the opportunity to generate, view and amend data presented within the findings to check authenticity and to further anonymise or generalise if they wished.

Participants attended an individual audio recorded interview. This was guided by certain themes: gaining a sense of the person; the impact of social work education on themselves; and the implications of this impact. This was followed by a one day group workshop where participants collaborated to develop representations of their experiences. This was through the use of objects, imagery, music, mind maps and verbal discussion. Within the course of the day, participants shared their own reflections and representations and encouraged and enabled each other to analyse and reflect on their experiences. They worked together to form the basis of a group representation in the form of a digital story (a series of visual images with an audio commentary). The story was further developed following the researcher-led workshop using their ideas and images and the words of the participants from their audio interviews. It was then shown to the participants to check accuracy and issues of anonymity but also as a catalyst for further analysis and reflection. It was then shared with other members of the participants' cohort for feedback on the meaning and resonance for them.

The Findings

The research findings include a range of materials and documents to present as close a picture as possible of the actual experience of the participants. The study did not seek to be representative of the cohort but to illuminate unique experiences. These are presented together to create a unitary appreciative profile (Cowling, 2004a, 2004b) of the impact of qualifying social work education on a person's beliefs, values and behaviour. The findings in relation to the participants' sense of well-being are summarised and presented within this paper as five individual profiles including the participants' own representations. Their perceptions and views are shared within the discussion.

Individual Profiles (Anonymised)

The Impact for Assad

Assad identifies himself as a black, Muslim, bi-lingual male with a multi-cultural background. His experience of social work education is characterised by significant challenges and changes to his own values and beliefs. He lives his life under the direction of his Muslim values but explains how many of his cultural beliefs were challenged through his learning on the social work degree. This in turn led him to question aspects of his culture and his own behaviour. Changes to his beliefs and values caused conflict for Assad with family and friends and within himself. His transition involved developing a value base that could be congruent to both his personal, religious, cultural and professional beliefs and values, which he feels he was successful in achieving. He believes that the emotional impact was negative at times but has had a positive outcome: 'I think (this course) is the best thing I have done. That's all I can say. I have learnt a lot. It's made a big difference'.

Assad chose a photo of his and a friend's hands on the Mission Impossible plaque on the walk of fame and his bike as representations of the impact on him of social work education.

> The hands are a photo of me and a friend I made on the course.
> It symbolises difference.
> The hands symbolise friendship.
> Mission impossible is how it feels sometimes.
> I used this bike to cycle to Uni everyday.
> The bike represents a journey.
> There are times when it's hard work going up hill.
> Sometimes it's a breeze, freewheeling down hill.
> Over the three years I have made changes and repaired parts.
> It has a new wheel.
> It's the same bike but its parts have changed.
> I'm the same person but I've adapted.

The Impact for Vicky

Vicky identifies herself as a white British female in her early twenties, from the North of England. She was 18 at the start of her social work education and she identifies herself as having changed a lot during this time. For her, the transition is one of becoming; becoming an adult, a professional, a social worker, a feminist. The transition has been influenced by moving away from home for the first time, becoming more independent, developing new friendships, experiencing difficulties with flat mates, becoming homeless for a short time, fleeing a threatening and potentially violent relationship and becoming more politically aware. The impact of this transition on Vicky's sense of well-being was substantial as she experienced many causes of instability over the three years and the gains came with many losses:

> I'll always love my friends and where I'm from but I hardly go back home now.
> I don't particularly feel at home there anymore and I didn't expect that to happen.
> I feel quite worried because I don't know what to do with myself now.

Vicky shared the same photo as Assad of their hands on the Mission Impossible plaque on the walk of fame and a 'thinking of you' card as representations of the impact on her of social work education.

> I spent my 21st birthday at home.
> There was a moment when I realised, I'd grown apart.
> I didn't really belong anymore.
> The card was from my Mum, "love you, miss you".
> It was significant that she needed to write a card.
> It was because I didn't go home as much.
> I chose the photo of the hands together with "Assad" when thinking about today.
> It's about new friendships.
> Accepting difference.

The Impact for Terry

Terry identifies himself as a 45-year-old, white British male, who is an atheist, has adopted what he feels are working class values as opposed to his parents middle class ones and who believes strongly in fairness, equity and that social justice is his core value. He reflects deeply on the impact of his childhood experiences on his beliefs, values and behaviour and on the impact of social work education in shaping these further. He feels that he has experienced change and provides examples of analysing his previous experiences and behaviours following particular areas of learning within the degree. This has had an impact on current relationships such as that with his father which has become more open. His sense of well-being was strengthened in many ways as he made sense of his past experiences and discovered a role and profession he felt he was good at. The process however was difficult:

> The learning experience as a whole has been really enjoyable. It sort of gives you resilience but it is so damned hard. It really is hard work. When you finish you'll think God have I earned this. It's going to be a bit of a personal milestone to me.

Terry chose a song: The Stranglers: *No More Heroes* and a Sully toy from the film Monsters Inc. as representations of the impact on him of social work education.

> I was a really huge Stranglers fan.
> There's a line, "Whatever happened to all the heroes?
> All the Shakespearoes, they watched their Rome burn.
> Whatever happened to all the heroes?"
> That would be my representation of the impact and knowing what I want to be.
> Sully lives in my car.
> When I'm driving kids when I'm at work, they can play with him.
> A kid I used to work with gave him to me, it was a gift.
> I saw him recently and was able to say I still had him.

I have a long drive into Uni from home.
I have spent a lot of time in the car. Sully is an unconditional listener.

The Impact for Jessica

Jessica identifies herself as a white British, able-bodied female in her early thirties. Her experience was influenced by the need to work full time throughout her three year degree and she describes feeling quite isolated at times from the year group and struggled to 'find her place'. She acknowledged the pressure she places on herself to do well and identified the impact of this stress, in particular from placement, on herself, her relationships and on her sense of well-being.

Jessica chose a clock, a diary and a 30th birthday card as representations of the impact on her of social work education.

Three years of diaries and a clock.
Everything is part of a schedule and is organised.
I find it quite comforting.
Knowing what I am going to be doing for the next year.
Having it all planned out.
It represents the need to juggle and manage everything.
I had a significant birthday and my niece was born.
I can think back to that day and I know what assignment I was working on.
I could only allow a short amount of time to celebrate.
I had to get back to my assignment.
I'm not sure about not knowing what's coming next.
I'm programmed now to work at this pace, I can't stop now!

The Impact for Linda

Linda identifies herself as female, Scottish British, and 42. Linda started the course with a strong sense of her identity and her values and a political interest and awareness. She didn't expect any huge changes to self during her social work education but believes that small changes have occurred. Change for her has been about becoming more open minded (and recognising that she wasn't as open minded as she had thought before), becoming more reflective and considered in her thinking and reflections and communicating more openly. She reflects on the impact this has had on her practice but also on her relationships and friendships: 'My friends think I'm more open, which can only be a good thing'.

Linda chose two albums: The Streets: *It was Supposed to be Easy* and Elbow: *Leaders of the Free World* as representations of the impact on her of social work education.

The Streets: *It was Supposed to be Easy.*
So much of this album is representative for me.
The title fits with how I feel.
The lyrics are a social commentary.
He lays it bare—is honest.
He thanks everyone who has ever "dissed" him for giving him focus.
I've listened to the Streets and Elbow so often during the three years.
It's become my soundtrack.

Discussion

All of the participants had experienced what Mezirow describes as perspective transformation or a change to their frame of reference, to one which is 'more inclusive, differentiating, permeable (open to other view points), critically reflective of assumptions, emotionally capable of change and integrative of experience' (Mezirow, 2000, p. 19 cited in Taylor, 2007). For all of the participants, this had, in part, impacted positively on their sense of well-being. They expressed feelings of confidence, self-belief, satisfaction and a feeling that their beliefs and behaviours were fair and just. There were many examples of challenging injustice and oppression, for example, which gave the participants a sense of satisfaction as well as examples of achievement gained through academic and professional success and which led to increased self-esteem.

The process of transition however—of becoming more aware, critically reflective of assumptions and open to other viewpoints—had led to some negative experiences and outcomes that affected their sense of well-being and quality of life. Participants described feelings of guilt, shame, frustration, anxiety, of losing a sense of belonging and identity, difficult family relationships, losing friendships and experiencing stressful situations. This was represented most strongly by the participants when expressing changes to their values and outlook and the impact on relationships with friends and family. Some of these experiences and the implications for their well-being are shared here.

Personal Values

The primary focus of the research study was to identify the impact on the students' lives of the focus of social work education to enable students to align their values with those of the profession. Linda and Jessica felt that their values had remained unchanged, due as they saw it to a congruence between their personal values and the professional ones they were encouraged to develop: 'I've retained most of my personal values and beliefs. My foundation is still the same. How I see things has changed'. As Jessica said: 'I think probably, before I would challenge things but now I challenge things and I have a better argument'. For them, the change had led them to feel more confident and assured in their own beliefs which satisfied a need for them and added to their sense of well-being.

Terry and Assad talked of how their value base changed as their knowledge and awareness increased. They both gave examples of this leading them to question old behaviour. As Terry said:

> There's this raft of knowledge about anti-racism that has really changed my value base. I had a few black friends at school but I'd be the first to say we used to be pretty abusive to each other. I want to go back and apologise to people to say sorry for what I've said. I feel ashamed and really guilty.

Assad also used his new learning to question old behaviours:

> My uncle I remember when I was young, now I understand that he was suffering from Schizophrenia but then, they said he had an evil spirit so nobody gave him any

> proper help or medication. They used to let him out in the sun all day. I regret that
> now, I wish I could challenge it. I did ask my Aunt one day, why did we treat him that
> way, he needed help. She doesn't have any answers.

The desire to go back and change previous actions was a common one amongst the participants which seemed to evidence the increase in awareness experienced by the participants as their new knowledge led them to reinterpret the meaning they had attached to previous experiences and events. For Terry and Assad, this desire formed part of their process of adjusting to a new awareness and knowledge. It caused uncomfortable feelings of shame and guilt for Terry and frustration and regret for Assad as they viewed their 'old selves' through the lens of the new. This created an inner conflict which affected their sense of well-being as they sought to adjust to their new outlook and make amends for their old behaviour. They both commented however on this change being for the better. The outcome impacted positively on their self-esteem and confidence which were key factors in maintaining a sense of well-being.

Relationships with Others

For all of the participants, shifts in their outlook, beliefs, values and behaviour had an impact on their relationships with others. All identified their relationships with friends or family as important to their sense of self and to their well-being and as a source of stability, support and identity. All however experienced changes to these relationships as a direct result of their social work education resulting in conflict, instability, disruption to social support networks and to their sense of identity and belonging.

Terry explained that his learning had led him to 'see oppression' everywhere and of the need to challenge this: 'People send you jokes and stuff and I had to say to my nephew last week, that's just bang out of order that is. Send me something funny, not that crap'. All of the participants talked of challenging friends, family and colleagues regarding what they felt to be discriminatory or oppressive comments. For Jessica with strong family support, this was accepted and she felt that her family had been open to the challenges and showed a willingness to 'get it right'. For Assad and Vicky, this had lost them friendships, in part due to their shifting values that meant they no longer wanted to spend time with certain people. As Vicky said, 'they hadn't changed, I had'. For Assad, it had caused difficulties in family relationships as his heightened awareness had caused him to question beliefs within his family:

> In my family my nephew said he was gay. Every member of the family was angry.
> I told them, it is his choice. They were not happy with me. Why are you supporting
> him? Why are you encouraging him? Including my own sister, she didn't talk to me
> for a while.

Vicky describes losing her sense of belonging. For her this led to significant feelings of instability and an unclear sense of who she was. It led to fewer visits home which also reduced her support networks which would ordinarily have maintained her sense of well-being. She links this with being less able to deal with difficulties which then presented during her time on the course but also as a factor in developing resilience, independence and maturity.

The impact had been stressful for all of those describing these experiences, a factor acknowledged by Collins *et al.* (2010) who comment on the transitional nature of professional courses being a likely factor in why social work and nursing students have been shown to have higher levels of stress than more traditional, non-vocational students. For all of the participants the impact on their relationships with friends, family and colleagues had resulted from shifts in their own beliefs and values but also their unwillingness to ignore comments, jokes and behaviour and their need to challenge oppression and discrimination when they saw it. Their social work education had affected not only their beliefs and values but also their behaviour outside of the classroom and the practice environment. All of them commented that their education had taught them to 'speak up'. What was striking about the impact expressed by the participants was that, despite some very difficult experiences and conflict (both internally and externally), this was buffered by the positive outcomes of their learning and a sense that their increased knowledge and understanding had 'made them a better person'. This view was supported by many of the participants' peers when sharing the representations created within the study with them. Despite stressful experiences and difficult periods of transition, all of the participants reported this to be a positive change but also a permanent one. As Assad commented, 'it's a long lasting change whether I like it or not!'.

Implications for Social Work Education

From my perspective, listening to the participants' stories and representations, I discovered many aspects of their lives and experiences that I had not known about which greatly increased my insight into their experiences, their processes of learning and their transition from student to professional. I concluded that it is important to recognise issues that have the potential to impact on a student's well-being, both in terms of our responsibility to provide a duty of care but also to enable them to make sense of their learning within the context of their own lives. It provides the opportunity to enable the students' learning to be in depth and meaningful by using their whole selves as a resource (Rogers, 1969; Knowles, 1984; Mezirow, 2000 cited in Taylor, 2007) but also in enabling them to adapt to these changes in a way that satisfies their needs and maintains a sense of well-being.

How we achieve this within social work education is perhaps at times assumed to be the domain of the practice placement and the role of the practice educator. The participants however argued that the focus should be as strong within university based education. One of the participants stated that she would have benefitted from one-to-one supervision within university based education rather than just on placement:

> The lecturer always said if I had any problems to come and see them but I've never really had any big problems. Placement is really good because you get to sit down with somebody and it may be a little thing but if it's not dealt with it can become a

big thing. It would have been nice to have had more time to just talk about your experiences and to reflect with someone else.

The challenge of social work educators is to develop strategies for students to satisfy this need within the available resources. Whilst practice learning support is key, the role of the university based educator is paramount in enabling student social workers to make sense of their learning in order to become the insightful, confident, resilient and empathic social workers the profession requires. It was important to the participants for educators to model these qualities.

In my own practice as an educator this has led to the exploration of a number of different approaches, some suggested by the participants and others as my response to the issues they raised. The next step will be to evaluate the effectiveness of these in supporting students with the transformative nature of social work education and in minimising the negative impact on their sense of well-being. These have or will include an increased focus within the curriculum across the year groups on preparing students for the potential impact; sharing strategies for dealing with stress and stressful situations; encouraging and supporting the development of peer support, mentoring and places to share experiences; and providing support for difficulties when needed. The goal of such strategies is not only to maintain the students' sense of well-being within social work education and as qualified social workers, but also to impact positively on their lives as a whole.

Conclusions

Whilst the research focussed on the unique experiences of just five participants, the aim of a unitary appreciative inquiry is to learn from these unique experiences to enhance our understanding of a particular context, in this case social work education. There are several conclusions that we can draw from the experiences represented in this paper that can inform our understanding of this impact. For the participants, there had certainly been an impact on their beliefs, values and behaviour as a result of their social work education. In most cases this was a process of increasing their awareness and opening their eyes to what was out there rather than fundamental changes. As Jessica said, 'I always used to challenge but now I can say because …' or as Vicky explained, she just hadn't realised the extent of certain issues. For Assad, some of his beliefs had fundamentally changed, such as beliefs regarding homosexuality and women's roles, as a result of being more open to other people's views and experiences. All of the participants talked of being more open, more empathic, more aware and having what Mezirow (2000 cited in Taylor, 2007) would describe as a more permeable frame of reference, having become more open to changes and challenges to their thinking.

For all of the participants however, this had impacted negatively on some of their relationships with friends and family and had led to internal conflict as they sought to adjust to their new ways of thinking and the implications for their behaviour both past and present. This had impacted negatively on their well-being as, for them, factors such as having a strong sense of identity, good support and social networks, stability, a sense of belonging and good relationships with others were key. The participants believed that whilst the process of change had at times been difficult and had impacted significantly on their lives, the outcome was positive. They felt that the difficult aspects of the transition were best supported within social work education when values and behaviours were modelled by staff, when educators acknowledged and understood the potential impact of their learning on themselves, and when networks for sharing experiences, seeking support and enabling slow, developmental change were available.

References

Argyris, C. & Schon, D. (1974) *Theory in Practice: Increasing Professional Effectiveness*, Jossey-Bass Classics, San Francisco, CA.

Coghlan, D. (2007) 'Insider action research doctorates: generating actionable knowledge', *Higher Education*, vol. 54, pp. 293–334.

Collins, S., Coffey, M. & Morris, L. (2010) 'Social work students: stress, support and well-being', *British Journal of Social Work*, vol. 40, no. 3, pp. 963–982.

Cowling, R. (2001) 'Unitary appreciative inquiry', *Advances in Nursing Science*, vol. 23, no. 4, pp. 32–38.

Cowling, R. (2004a) 'Pattern, participation, praxis and power in unitary appreciative nursing perspective', *Advances in Nursing Science*, vol. 27, no. 3, pp. 202–214.

Cowling, R. (2004b) 'Despair: a unitary appreciative inquiry', *Advances in Nursing Science*, vol. 27, no. 4, pp. 287–300.

Cowling, R. (2005) 'Despairing women and healing outcomes: a unitary appreciative inquiry', *Advances in Nursing Science*, vol. 27, no. 4, pp. 287–300.

Darra, S. (2008) 'Emotion work and ethics of novice insider research', *Journal of Research in Nursing*, vol. 13, pp. 251–261.

Fook, J. (2004) 'Critical reflection and transformative possibilities', in *Social Work in a Corporate Era*, eds L. Davies & P. Leonard, Ashgate, Aldershot.

Gardner, F. (2001) 'Social work students and self awareness: how does it happen?', *Reflective Practice*, vol. 2, no. 1, pp. 27–40.

Gould, N. & Baldwin, M. (2004) *Social Work, Critical Reflection and the Learning Organisation*, Ashgate, Aldershot.

Green Lister, P. (2003) '"It's like you can't be a whole person, a mother who studies." Lifelong learning: mature women students with caring commitments in social work education', *Social Work Education*, vol. 22, no. 2, pp. 125–138.

Gunasekara, C. (2007) 'Pivoting the centre: reflections on undertaking qualitative interviewing in academia', *Qualitative Research*, vol. 7, pp. 461–475.

Hafford-Letchfield, T. (2007) 'Factors affecting retention of learners following a degree in social work at a university in the South East of England', *Learning in Health and Social Care*, vol. 6, no. 3, pp. 170–184.

Johns, C. (2005) 'Dwelling with Alison: a reflection on expertise', *Complimentary Therapies in Clinical Practice*, vol. 11, pp. 37–44.

Kamya, H. (2000) 'Hardiness and spirituality among social work students: implications for social work education', *Journal of Social Work Education*, vol. 36, no. 2, pp. 234–240.

Knowles, M. (1984) *The Adult Learner: A Neglected Species*. 3rd edn. Gulf Publishing, Houston, TX.

Lord Laming (2003) *The Victoria Climbie Inquiry Report of an Inquiry by Lord Laming* [online]. Available at: www.dh.gov.uk/en/Publicationsandstatistics/.../DH-4008654.

Lord Laming (2009) *Protection of Children in England: A Progress Report* [online]. Available at: www.publications.education.gov.uk/eOrderingDownload/HC-330.pdf.

Malone, S. (2003) 'Ethics at home: informed consent in your own backyard', *Qualitative Studies in Education*, vol. 16, no. 6, pp. 797–815.

Mercer, J. (2007) 'The challenges of insider research in educational institutions: wielding a double-edged sword and resolving delicate dilemmas' *Oxford Review of Education*, vol. 33, no. 1, pp. 1–17.

Mezirow, J. (1996) 'Contemporary paradigms of learning', *Adult Education Quarterly*, vol. 46, no. 3, pp. 158–172.

Miller, W. L. & Crabtree, B.F. (1999) 'Depth interviewing', in *Doing Qualitative Research*, eds B. F. Crabtree & W. L. Miller. 2nd edn. Sage, London.

Pardeck, J. T. & McCallister, R. L. (1991) 'The effects of undergraduate social work education on the personal growth and development of students', *Social Work Education*, vol. 11, pp. 382–387.

Reupert, A. (2007) 'Social worker's use of self', *Clinical Social Work Journal*, no. 35, pp. 107–116.

Rogers, C. R. (1969) *Freedom to Learn: A View of What Education Might Become*, Columbus, OH: Charles Merrill.

Skills for Care (2002) *Statement of Expectations of People Using Services and Their Carers* [online]. Available at: http://www.niscc.info/content/uploads/downloads/workforce_dev/NOS_health_social/Statement_expectations.pdf.

Social Work Taskforce (2009) *Final Report of the Social Work Taskforce* [online]. Available at: www.dcsf.gov.uk/swtf.

Taylor, E. (2007) 'An update of transformative learning theory: a critical review of the empirical research (1999–2005)', *International Journal of Lifelong Education*, vol. 26, pp. 173–191.

TOPSS UK Partnership (2002) *National Occupational Standards for Social Work* [online]. Available at: http://www.skillsforcare.org.uk/developing_skills/National_Occupational_Standards/social_work.aspx, accessed 15 February 2010.

White, S., Fook, J. & Gardner, F. (2006) *Critical Reflection in Health and Social Care*, McGraw Hill, Maidenhead, Berkshire.

World Health Organisation (WHO) (1986) 'The Ottawa Charter for health promotion', *First International Conference on Health Promotion*, Ottawa, 21 November 1986 [online]. Available at: http://www.who.int/healthpromotion/conferences/previous/ottawa/en/index.html, accessed 20 September 2010.

Older Women and Craft: Extending Educational Horizons in Considering Wellbeing

Jane Maidment & Selma Macfarlane

While the social work literature is broader and more holistic than many disciplines, we undoubtedly still limit the knowledge we draw upon in ways that stifle our creativity in conceptualising and attempting to facilitate wellbeing, which flows on to limit our teaching. In particular, the significance to wellbeing of place and social space, the value of informal networks to generate support and opportunities for reciprocity, and the inherent therapeutic value of creative activity appears to be neglected. In this paper we draw upon a small Australian research study around older women and craftmaking to explore how learning from diverse disciplines, such as critical gerontology and textile making, can illuminate our understanding of wellbeing. We relate this discussion to examining notions of ageing that go beyond a focus on illness and deterioration, to enhance positive and diverse concepts of health in the context of everyday life. We then discuss the implications for social work education, with particular emphasis on ageing, and argue that by engaging with a diverse range of disciplines, we are able to think about, teach and advocate for wellbeing in more expansive and useful ways.

Introduction: Re-evaluating the Social Work Knowledge Base

There is ready acknowledgement in the social work literature attesting to the rapidly changing practice and policy context, increased workloads and complexity of client issues being encountered by workers (Baines, 2006). These trends, together with emergent areas of concern impacting upon community health, including social, technological, and environmental sustainability (Zapf, 2009), raise questions about the efficacy of traditional social work education for preparing future practitioners. In a recently published call for action, social work has been dared to foster 'education that is capable of challenging existing paradigms, critically evaluating emerging alternatives, and encouraging action grounded in new ways of understanding the world' (Jones, 2010, p. 68). This robust appeal to the profession warrants a serious examination of our existing knowledge base, and consideration of how we might strengthen our capacity to meet emerging practice challenges in order to strengthen individual and community health and wellbeing.

Social work education and practice has traditionally been embedded within an understanding and application of theory and method derived from a range of sources. These sources have been variously described using discipline based categorisations, such as psychology, sociology, anthropology, economics, politics, law, medicine and the social sciences (Chenoweth and McAuliffe, 2005). The diversity of knowledge influences on practice have been simultaneously criticised for being incoherent and conceptually untidy (Clark, 2008, p. 44), and praised for their holistic and dynamic nature.

Nevertheless, paradigm shifts in the way people live their lives prompted by the impacts of globalisation necessitate a re-examination of the knowledge base that informs social work and the way it is practised. The emergence of global ageing, the exponential growth in geographic mobility of kith and kin, rapidly changing technologies and environmental estrangement require practitioners to engage with an expanded understanding of ecological knowledge and awareness (Jones, 2010), a deepened sense of the spiritual influences on wellbeing, in conjunction with overt political activism (Besthorn, 2003). In the interests of promoting strategies to nurture sustainable individual and community wellbeing, connections between social work and a broader content and process knowledge base is warranted. These efforts to think and engage more generally across diverse sources of knowledge and insight also need to be reflected in our social work curriculum and continuing professional education.

Using research conducted with nine women in Victoria, Australia we demonstrate how connecting with principles related to social sustainability within creative design can potentially enhance practice interventions with older people. This work is underpinned by recognition of the centrality of *interdependence* between those working in diverse disciplines, between practitioners and clients, between community and business interests, and between older people themselves, to generate innovative living, helping and educating synergies. For social work, moving beyond consideration of wellbeing within a strictly health focused paradigm signals a readiness to communicate and promote education not only between health related disciplines but together with practitioners, volunteers and laypeople in quite different fields. The rationale for such an approach can be found in Popper's assertion that, 'We are not students of some subject matter, but students of problems. And problems may cut right across the borders of any subject matter or discipline' (Popper, 1963, p. 88). While Popper's 'problem' focused discourse does not particularly resonate with social work, recognising the potential for diverse parties with different forms of expertise to contribute to solution building is generally a supported tenet in this discipline (Saleeby and Day, 2008). With this principle in mind it has been argued that there is always the potential for substantial omission (of understanding) if issues based knowledge is wholly constructed within specific disciplines (Campbell, 1969 cited in Ellis, 2008, p. 8). To this end we argue that social work practice with older people will be strengthened through interdisciplinary educational inquiry and intervention, where students discover not simply the content contribution that diverse disciplines make to shaping wellbeing, but learn the skills and processes for crossing ontological and epistemological borders, making this type of collaboration a practice reality. Our work with older craftswomen in Victoria has demonstrated to us that the liminal thresholds 'betwixt and between' disciplines (Ellis, 2008), offer up unexplored territories and significant potential for promoting wellbeing amongst older people.

Not surprisingly, this conceptualisation of what might be 'relevant' information for practice prompts reconsideration of the relationship between power and knowledge, the potential for some migration of specialisms, with the hybridisation of knowledge development between disciplines being inevitable (Ellis, 2008, p. 11). Subsequent implications for breaking down the existing knowledge silos for social work practice and education are discussed in more depth later in this article. Suffice at this stage to signal that a re-examination of this order necessitates engagement with notions of critical pedagogy. Critical pedagogy, according to McArthur (2010, p. 301) 'has a strong commitment to interdisciplinarity, [regarding] interdisciplinary spaces as crucial to the pursuit of emancipatory ideals', and thus vital to higher education's wider social purpose to create 'changes in society in the direction of social justice' (McLean, 2006 cited in McArthur, 2010, pp. 302–303). These wider aims for higher education clearly resonate with social work education and practice.

Craft, Wellbeing and Ageing

Systematic attempts to research subjective wellbeing in conjunction with the engagement with art and craft have been limited (Reynolds, 2010, p. 135). This lack of attention to the contribution that creative endeavours make towards fostering personal health is evidenced through a review of 1,085 articles within the first 65 volumes of *Social Indicators Research* where not one publication documented the impact of participation in the arts on wellbeing (Michalos, 2005, p. 12). Further indications of inattention to the relationship between the arts and wellbeing is reflected in the social work literature, where a review of the last 10 years of publication records in six prominent social work journals (*Australian Social Work*; *British Journal of Social Work*; *Social Work Education*; *Families in Society*; *Canadian Journal of Social Work*; *International Social Work*) found just seven articles exploring participation in arts and crafts in association with social work practice and research. As such the connection between fostering wellbeing with participation in arts and craft is rarely acknowledged in social work, despite reminders in the professional literature that creativity has positive associations with wellbeing, health and life satisfaction

(Grace *et al.*, 2009, p. 241), with artistic expression being associated with strengthening identity, building resilience and facilitating solace and healing (Crisp, 2010).

As social work educators and practitioners we recognise that we bring not only professional knowledge to our work, but also our personal, multi-faceted selves. Our own experiences of wellbeing stem from many sources and are part of our identities. For those of us who are craftswomen, we carry this involvement—or even passion— with us; in the same way, other social workers who are musicians or writers or walkers bring these aspects of their identity and wellbeing to their work. While we may consider these pastimes and creative endeavours to be therapeutic, empowering and enriching in our own lives, it seems we have not adequately acknowledged their beneficial nature in the lives of others, particularly those labelled as 'clients'. Most of us did not study such things as part of our social work education; in fact, while notions of illness, oppression and disempowerment were addressed, the notion of 'wellbeing' in a more holistic and creative sense has been widely neglected in traditional social work education. We therefore draw upon the textile and crafting literature to illustrate how creative endeavours may be used to promote wellbeing.

Craft has been identified as an item that fulfils a function, requires the use of the hands to create and uses materials identified as natural—something both functional and aesthetically pleasing (MacEachren, 2004). Historically, textile handcrafting was entwined with women's history: work done in the private sphere that was relatively child safe and could be picked up and put down—'the most visible result of women's labour [providing] tangible lasting proof of a woman's skills' (Johnson and Wilson, 2005, p. 115). Despite many viable alternatives available today, handcrafts have not disappeared (Johnson and Wilson, 2005).

Engagement with craft provides an experience that 'balances and unifies the needs of both mind and body' (MacEachren, 2004, p. 143). Csikszentmihalyi (1990 cited in Reynolds, 2010, p. 136) suggests that 'serious leisure activities'—those that invite challenge and commitment—are linked with the experience of 'flow', which describes 'an experience of deep engagement'. This feeling of engagement or interest is an emotion that is both a form of wellbeing in itself, and one that may lead to other forms of wellbeing such as the development of diverse life experiences and skills (Dik and Hansen, 2008). Textile handcrafting has also been described as a means of dealing particularly with health related issues as well as stressful situations of daily life, promoting mental health, while 'forging an alternative identity to that of being a sick person' (Gandolfo and Grace, 2009, p. 16). Reynolds (2010, p. 138), in her study of how visual art-making (including craft and painting) contributed to the subjective wellbeing of older women in the UK, found that the women valued art-making for 'its capacity to stimulate thought and learning', and the way everyday life was enriched by 'sensuous experiences, challenges, playful experiments, and the pleasure of developing new skills and expertise'.

Contemporary women crafters affirm that craft contributes to their sense of a meaningful identity, as they realise their individual goals and creative aspirations (Schofield-Tomschin and Littrell, 2001), and leave a trail of artefacts that affirm the role they have with family and friends (Johnson and Wilson, 2005). Art-making as a process can be particularly important in protecting older women's self-identities, which may suffer due to ageist stereotyping and exclusionary social practices (Schofield-Tomschin and Littrell, 2001; Reynolds, 2010). As such the experience of vulnerability and frailty that older women may experience can co-exist with wisdom, resilience and affirmation (Gattuso, 2003).

In addition to being useful and unique, 'textile objects communicate meanings to producers and owners' (Schofield-Tomschin and Littrell, 2001, p. 42). 'Mastering the skills to make a useful item allows the maker to offer to others the "gifts" embedded in the made item'—for example the warmth of socks (MacEachren, 2004, p. 145). Making an item that is useful to another is a form of serving or sharing that encourages a sense of citizenship while contributing to community wellbeing (MacEachren, 2004), often across generations. The importance of *reciprocity*, as suggested here, resonates with notions of connection, contribution and attachment to community, bringing with it a sense of generativity and meaning in life (Craft and Grasser, 1998).

Our own research into the relationship between craft and wellbeing amongst older women demonstrates engagement with these activities is often associated with fostering experiential forms of learning in supportive peer learning environments (Maidment and Macfarlane, 2008), where opportunities exist for increasing social networks and relationship building (Schofield-Tomschin and Littrell, 2001; Johnson and Wilson, 2005). Schofield-Tomschin and Littrell (2001) observe that 'women bind themselves symbolically to other women by their membership in small social groups' (2001, p. 41). At a time of life when friendship may become more difficult to maintain, 'natural' network groups—those based on common interests—can contribute significantly to combating loneliness, decreasing isolation and enhancing wellbeing in older age (Stevens, 2001), with recent research noting that due to geographic mobility and changing employment patterns older people are more likely to depend upon their own 'personal community' rather than kin to provide companionship (Gray, 2009, p. 8). In conjunction with these observations the sustaining protective and restorative health functions of sturdy friendships are well documented in recent research (Cummins and Mead, 2008), as is the capacity for craft groups to provide the infrastructure to foster these strong friendship networks (Maidment and Macfarlane, 2008).

Research Method and Design

The initial premise on which we developed our pilot research included the position statement that participation by older women with informal craft activities could ameliorate the need for engagement with formal social services. The focus for this inquiry grew out of recognition that social connection and subjective wellbeing appear to provide protective effects against ill-health and mortality in the aged (Malta, 2005; Reynolds, 2010), while at the same time noting that the impact of participation in the arts on wellbeing has been comprehensively ignored (Michalos, 2005). Given our own observations of the large numbers of older women participating in some form of craft venture we were curious to explore the curative, restorative and protective factors these activities appeared to offer.

The *literature review* for this research took us as social workers into the hitherto unfamiliar disciplines of textile design, as discussed above (Schofield-Tomschin and Littrell, 2001) and micro geographies (Wiles *et al.*, 2008), where the concepts of place, space and belonging, nurturing creativity and meaning making provide diverse explanations on factors that promote wellbeing. As such our pilot research with older craftswomen provides an example of crossing the traditional knowledge thresholds which inform social work, creating new possibilities for imaginative and sustainable social work intervention in the field of ageing.

The *method* for conducting the research included semi-structured interviews with nine women aged between 54 and 86. The 54-year-old in this sample was a daughter of one of the older participants and as such was the youngest of those interviewed by 16 years. The remaining eight participants were aged between 70 and 84 years of age. The participant craftswomen were sourced from two craft groups in a regional town based in Victoria, Australia. These women volunteered to be interviewed after hearing a presentation about the research, its purpose and process from the authors. Prior to conducting the interviews late in 2007 and early 2008, an ethics application was submitted and subsequently approved by the Deakin University Ethics Committee. Given the regional site for this study, particular care needed to be taken to ensure that the identity of individual participants was protected. To this end all results have been reported using pseudonyms with other unique identifying information offered during the interviews being removed.

Participants were provided with examples of the questions prior to conducting the interviews in order to have a sense of the sorts of information being sought. Examples of these questions include 'What do you get out of being involved in craftwork?' and 'To what extent (if any) does craftwork contribute to your own sense of wellbeing?'. The interviews lasted between 45 minutes and two hours. They were audio-recorded, transcribed and then organised using Nvivo. The data were subsequently coded and analysed independently by two of the researchers. While the scope and focus of this article does not provide an opportunity for comprehensive feedback on the analysis procedure and specific results [and these can be found in publications elsewhere (Maidment and Macfarlane, 2008, 2011)], the trends indicated in the findings suggest that social work educators and practitioners have much to learn about the wellbeing, expression of autonomy and personal agency of older people through engaging with discourses commonly found in creative arts. These include taking cognisance of:

- *The sustenance gained from being amidst creative endeavour, colour and textiles...*

  I have a few health problems and sometimes you get up and think I feel terrible today and you can go really down when you feel like that, when your bits and pieces hurt, I feel bad today and then I think to myself I can't do this to myself, so I'd be better off sewing, and I have a love of materials, and might spend an hour sorting out materials and before I know it I am right into it ... (Betty)

  You might go to find the tiniest little piece of material you remember you have for something so you have to go through this great big ... cane basket, and it's full ... and you never throw away any little bits, and you go scrounging through for leaf material or something like that, and even at home you are occupied even if you don't do a lot of craft you are thinking I had some material I could have done a rose or something like that. (Ruby)

- *The use of arts and craft as a vehicle for bringing potentially isolated groups of people together, generating ongoing friendships and staying connected with others*

Some days, we didn't do anything, we just sat there and laughed. We never put pressure on ourselves to have anything done. It's a matter of getting together and spending a day like women do ... swap the odd recipe and talk about the grandchildren, and ... if anything is wrong. (Elizabeth)

One of our ladies is 86 and she doesn't drive ... so she's picked up and brought here or wherever we are going. (Ruby)

A lot of the girls who started out as loners have now formed friendships in that group and quite often they go to patchwork shops together and have been able to mingle and form new friendships ... meeting all these new people all different personalities, but with the same love of what we're doing. (Elsie)

- *The sense of pride, accomplishment and confidence gained from having made an artefact, learned or taught a new crafting technique ...*

I love it when someone asks you, "how did you do that?" ... and I say, "if you do this and that" ... and you feel, I don't know, a bit important. (Elsie)

I think if you're learning something—and at my age in the mid 70s you think you've learned all you can—but there is always another thing to get enthused about ... I enjoy helping people to learn things because I've got so much out of it myself. (Betty)

- *The generative and healing nature of long standing naturally occurring communities of interest ...*

We are all in our seventies and we've all enjoyed such a long, long time together. (Ruby)

I get to meet people I get to be in company with other ladies, and I enjoy doing it. I get a bit lonely ... so it's good for me to go out and be with great people. (Helene)

- *Using craft activities to provide a sense of purpose and meaning in life through contributing to the community and wellbeing of others ...*

Whatever we are doing is now helping Red Cross because the sale of what we make goes to help other countries ... all the appeals, we are helping the Mongolian children at the moment ... if there's any disasters whatever we make goes straight into that, but Mongolia was the last project. (Ruby)

This is my outlet to be in the free time, to do things for others ... I like to think I can help somewhere, and when it's been long since you've worked, you can't give money to charity. But you can provide by doing this work that you like and enjoy ... and that is a great lift then—how I feel myself, knowing I am helping someone. (Betty)

- *Use of craft to affirm identity and place in the world ...*

... we were talking about it and he said to me "If you die while you're in surgery what will I do with all your quilts?", because I have some 60 or 70 down there. I said

"Don't worry about them just wrap me up in them, I'm going to be cremated, you can do that and won't have to buy a coffin". So the next day when I went to (the group) I was telling them, "Bill (not his real name) is worried I'm going to die so I told me to wrap me up in the quilts". "Oh don't do that! Tell him to put in the paper all those attending the service will receive a quilt then you'll be sure of getting an audience!!". (Betty)

It's craft with a purpose ... older women now have got the chance to participate in so much more than they used to be able to, because once they outlived the usefulness of being a grandmother when the grandkids grew up, and weren't needed any more, so they sat down and become un-needed. (Thelma)

- *The benefits of experiencing what Csikszentmihalyi (1990 cited in Reynolds, 2010) described as the 'flow' ...*

I get involved and with the work that I do I am not thinking of other bad things ... you concentrate and forget, you forget what you're worried about. (Helene)

The passages above illustrate in a small way the multiple benefits to health and wellbeing that the older women we interviewed experienced through being part of a craft group. As educators we were struck with how a low cost intervention, such as linking a person interested in arts and crafts with such a group, could have a powerful flow-on effect, in terms of building and sustaining self-esteem and community connectedness. While this observation may seem self-evident, on examining our social work educational curriculum and professional literature we were struck by the absence of acknowledgment given to the arts as a means of kindling self-worth, meaningful social roles and active community participation. Through completing this research we discovered the liminal spaces between social work and textile design which helped us to conceptualise new understandings and ways for promoting health and wellbeing in social work practice with older people.

Reconfiguring Social Work Education?

Oversight in the area of the arts and wellbeing has prompted us to question the sorts of knowledge considered as 'legitimate' for inclusion in social work education curriculum and discourse. This questioning led us into the territory of the liminal spaces between social work and the disciplines of the arts and textile design and, while not specifically discussed in this article, we were also challenged during the research to consider knowledge dimensions associated with architecture, urban planning and technology studies in terms of the way these discourses impacted upon the women's craft activities. From our research and own experiences as craftswomen we argue that testing and reconfiguring disciplinary pedagogical boundaries to include consider-ation of disciplines as diverse as creative arts, are likely to open up new empowering ways to work with people and communities. The development of a new lens through which to explore human functioning and potential contributes to the ongoing evolution of social work practice, within an expanded understanding of ecological knowledge and awareness (Jones, 2010).

Social work's commitment to respond to everyday human problems across a wide spectrum of practice fields is a hallmark of the profession. Students in professionally qualifying social work courses study a range of subjects from various disciplines including politics, health and sociology, exemplifying awareness of the multi-faceted nature of individual and social life. Social work students develop skills in critical analysis, critical reflection and working across boundaries; hence, students, educators and practitioners are potentially ideally placed to embrace diverse sources of knowledge, whether from other disciplines or outside traditional 'disciplinary' categories altogether, in the interests of fostering individual wellbeing and the creation of a more socially just society.

At the same time, over the four years of their course, social work students develop a strong sense of themselves as belonging to a unique professional group, and that 'to be engaged in a discipline is to shape, and be shaped by, the subject, to be part of a scholarly community, to engage with fellow students—to become "disciplined"' (Parker, 2010, p. 374). Social work is constantly evolving, and while drawing from a strong theory, value and skill base, is 'modelled not as a citadel ... guarded by experts, but as a community of practitioners', taught by educators who believe in and communicate the importance of their discipline, whilst engaging in a reflective, dialogical and critical approach (Parker, 2010, p. 379). This approach includes a commitment to social change, by moving beyond the capacity to think and reflect critically 'to actively frame problems or issues in a way that points out the road to transformative change' (McArdle and Mansfield, 2007, p. 496). This willingness to reframe problems or issues enables us as educators to productively deconstruct professional discourses and examine the positions that social workers occupy within them. Our expertise, as social workers and social work educators, may be enhanced by our ability to listen and look for opportunities to step outside disciplinary boundaries: to 'trade in ideas by transgressing discursive frontiers', recognising that ideas impact on both the individuals we work with, as well as having resonance within the wider socio-political context (hooks and West, 1991 cited in McLaren, 1996, p. 137).

By listening to the group of older craftswomen, we developed a better understanding of the role that craftmaking, community belonging and interconnect-edness had in relation to fostering individual wellbeing. At the same time we were encouraged to recognise the importance of advocating for the provision of creative meeting spaces for all community members, and developing imaginative ways in which the needs of older people are interwoven into a range of opportunities that provide genuine and empowering choices for people as they age.

Disciplines then, can be seen and experienced not so much as 'demarcations but communities ... with fluid structures based on common concerns' (Parker, 2010, p. 381). Students can be encouraged to engage, not simply with curriculum content, but with the 'processes of knowledge production ... asking questions about the nature of the knowledge [needed] in order to engage with and practise the discipline' (Parker, 2010, pp. 381–382). This 'critical professionalism' can be enhanced by strategies that promote *interdependence* in higher education (Davidson, 2004, p. 299). For educators, this process involves decentering the academic self by acknowledging that there are diverse ways of knowing the world, critically engaging with the wider purposes of (disciplinary-based) work, and looking over 'the hedges surrounding our own discipline' (Davidson, 2004, p. 305). This pursuit does not require the abandonment of one's own 'academic tribe and territory', but involves working collaboratively to explore issues across disciplines (Davidson, 2004, p. 310). We learned this lesson through conducting our research with older women engaged in crafting, where we discovered paradigms more commonly associated with creativity, art and design have much to offer our professional understanding of personal and community wellbeing. Our experience in this research affirms the claim that if social work educators have a responsibility to 'be leaders in building a society where human worth is not defined in monetary terms' (Wehbi and Turcotte, 2007, pp. 3–6) we need to draw on an even wider range of thought and experience, to ensure that deeper explanations of social problems and their potential remedies are not jettisoned in favour of superficial explanations, primarily aimed more at management and control rather than empowerment and wellbeing (Ferguson, 2008, p 19, citing Howe, 1996). This focus is particularly important in relation to our aged population, whose worth and contribution to community and wider society is often devalued.

Adopting *critical interdisciplinarity* then, can potentially help defend the complexity of higher education (McArthur, 2010, pp. 302–303) and return disciplines to their rightful place for 'develop[ing] minds to contribute to understanding and knowing how to act in the world', balancing critique and imagination, while acknowledging the permeable and dynamic nature of disciplinary communities. We are mindful that in this process it is not only higher education that is complex. So too is the rapidly changing world in which practitioners are engaged, necessitating increasingly open minds and imaginations to educate the social workers of the future.

The capacity for social work educators and practitioners to make connections across boundaries—disciplinary, paradigmatic, cultural, organisational or group—requires skills in developing deep and genuine knowledge through active curiosity, imaginatively seeking commonalities and interconnections, perceiving and building on strengths, and using power and influence wisely (Adams, 2005, p. 112). By encouraging students to engage in critical reflection and to consider 'transformational best case scenarios', educators can assist students to develop a willingness to reconsider practice and embrace new ideas and interdependence in responding to 'the diversity and full extent of people's needs' (Adams, 2005, p. 114). For the older women we talked with, interdependence between the members in their groups, and between the women and the wider community they contributed their craft to, was crucial to their wellbeing.

In relation to social work curricula itself, educators can continue to focus on both micro and macro levels of practice, acknowledging the significance of community and place, creativity, connectedness and wellbeing for diverse members in the community. This may involve policy advocacy for greater public investment by government in creative and art-related projects across the lifespan; promotion of well-designed urban and non-urban landscapes that cater to all—young, old and in-between; and the creation of community spaces that encourage diverse forms of citizenship and participation. More specifically, social work courses need to re-visit the place of 'the aged' in their curriculum, as this field of practice continues to be as invisible and marginalised as elders themselves (Hughes and Heycox, 2010), with even feminist literature having neglected to focus on old women, aging, and the political nature of age relations (Calasanti *et al.*, 2006).

Fostering health and wellbeing amongst a growing ageing population will require flexible, imaginative and transformational approaches, that encourage connectedness and acknowledge interdependence between older people themselves as well as those working in the caring professions. This approach will require social work educators to extend current discipline-specific educational horizons beyond the grand narratives to include voices from the margins. We argue in this article for educators to shift their pedagogical gaze to include wisdom from the creative arts and textile design when attempting to help students understand the notions of health and wellbeing.

References

Adams, R. (2005) 'Working within and across boundaries: tensions and dilemmas', in *Social Work Futures: Crossing Boundaries, Transforming Practice*, eds R. Adams, L. Dominelli & M. Payne, Palgrave Macmillan, Basingstoke, pp. 99–114.

Baines, D. (2006) '"If you could change one thing": social service workers and restructuring', *Australian Social Work*, vol. 59, no. 1, pp. 20–34.

Besthorn, F. H. (2003) 'Radical ecologisms: insights for educating social workers in ecological activism and social justice', *Critical Social Work: An Interdisciplinary Journal*, vol. 3, no. 1, pp. 66–106.

Calasanti, T., Slevin, K. & King, N. (2006) 'Ageism and feminism: from "et cetera" to center', *National Women's Studies Association Journal*, vol. 18, no. 1, pp. 13–30.

Chenoweth, L. & McAuliffe, D. (2005) *The Road to Social Work & Human Service Practice*, Thomson, Southbank.

Clark, J. (2008) 'Complex approaches to wicked problems: applying Sharon Berlin's analysis of dichotomous thinking', *Social Work Now: The Practice Journal of Child, Youth and Family*, vol. 39, pp. 38–48.

Craft, B. & Grasser, C. (1998) 'The relationship of reciprocity to self health care of older women', *Journal of Women & Ageing*, vol. 10, no. 2, pp. 35–47.

Crisp, B. (2010) *Spirituality and Social Work*, Ashgate, Burlington, VT.

Cummins, R. & Mead, R. (2008) *What Makes Us Happy?* Australian Unity Wellbeing Index, Survey 18, Report 18.2, Australian Unity, Deakin University, Melbourne.

Davidson, M. (2004) 'Bones of contention: using self and story in the quest to professionalize higher education teaching—an interdisciplinary approach', *Teaching in Higher Education*, vol. 9, no. 3, pp. 299–310.

Dik, B. & Hansen, J. (2008) 'Following passionate interests to well-being', *Journal of Career Assessment*, vol. 16, no. 1, pp. 86–100.

Ellis, R. (2008) 'Problems may cut across the borders. Why we cannot do without interdisciplinarity', in *Interdisciplinary Learning and Teaching in Higher Education*, eds B. Chandramohan & S. Fallows, Routledge, Hoboken.

Ferguson, I. (2008) *Reclaiming Social Work: Challenging Neo-liberalism and Promoting Social Justice*, SAGE Publications, London.

Gandolfo, E. & Grace, M. (2009) ... *It Keeps Me Sane ... Women Craft Wellbeing*, The Vulgar Press, Spotlight, Victoria University, Melbourne.

Gattuso, S. (2003) 'Becoming a wise old woman: resilience and wellness in later life', *Health Sociology Review*, vol. 12, no. 2, pp. 171–177.

Grace, M., Gandolfo, E. & Candy, C. (2009) 'Crafting quality of life. Creativity and wellbeing', *Journal of Association for Research on Mothering*, vol. 11, no. 1, pp. 239–250.

Gray, A. (2009) 'The social capital of older people', *Ageing and Society*, vol. 29, pp. 5–31.

Hughes, M. & Heycox, K. (2010) *Older People Ageing and Social Work: Knowledge for Practice*, Allen & Unwin, Crows Nest, NSW.

Johnson, J. & Wilson, L. (2005) 'It says you really care: motivational factors of contemporary female handcrafters', *Clothing & Textiles Research Journal*, vol. 23, no. 2, pp. 115–130.

Jones, P. (2010) 'Responding to the ecological crisis: transformative pathways for social work education', *Journal of Social Work Education*, vol. 46, no. 1, pp. 67–84.

MacEachren, Z. (2004) 'Function and aesthetics: defining craftsmanship', *Journal of Experiential Education*, vol. 26, no. 3, pp. 138–151.

Maidment, J. & Macfarlane, S. (2008) 'Craft groups: sites of friendship, empowerment, belonging and learning for older women', *Groupwork*, vol. 19, no. 1, pp. 10–25.

Maidment, J. & Macfarlane, S. (2011) 'Crafting communities: promoting inclusion, empowerment and learning between older women', *Australian Social Work*. DOI: 10.1080/0312407X.2010.520087.

Malta, S. (2005) *Social Connectedness and Health Amongst Older Adults*, TASA Conference, University of Tasmania, 6–8 December.

McArdle, K. & Mansfield, S. (2007) 'Voice, discourse and transformation: enabling learning for the achieving of social change', *Discourse: Studies in the Cultural Politics of Education*, vol. 28, no. 4, pp. 485–498.

McArthur, J. (2010) 'Time to look anew: critical pedagogy and disciplines within higher education', *Studies in Higher Education*, vol. 35, no. 3, pp. 301–315.

McLaren, P. (1996) 'Liberatory politics and higher education: a Frierean perspective', in *Counternarratives: Cultural Studies and Critical Pedagogies in Postmodern Spaces*, eds H. Giroux, C. Lankshear, P. McLaren & M. Peters, Routledge, New York & London, pp. 117–148.

Michalos, A. (2005) 'Arts and the quality of life: an exploratory study', *Social Indicators Research*, vol. 71, pp. 11–59.

Parker, J. (2010) 'A new disciplinarity: communities of knowledge, learning and practice', *Teaching in Higher Education*, vol. 7, no. 4, pp. 373–386.

Popper, K. (1963) *Conjectures and Refutations: The Growth of Scientific Knowledge*, Routledge and Kegan Paul, New York.

Reynolds, F. (2010) '"Colour and communion": exploring the influences of visual art-making as a leisure activity on older women's subjective well-being', *Journal of Aging Studies*, vol. 24, pp. 135–143.

Saleeby, D. & Day, P (2008) *The Strengths Perspective in Social Work Practice*. 5th edn. Allyn & Bacon Inc, Boston, MA.

Schofield-Tomschin, S. & Littrell, M. (2001) 'Textile handcraft guild participation: a conduit to successful aging', *Clothing and Textiles Research Journal*, vol. 19, no. 2, pp. 41–51.

Stevens, N. (2001) 'Combating loneliness: a friendship enrichment programme for older women', *Ageing and Society*, vol. 21, pp. 183–202.

Wehbi, S. & Turcotte, P. (2007) 'Social work education: neoliberalisms' willing victim?', *Critical Social Work*, vol. 8, no. 1.

Wiles, J., Allen, R., Palmer, A., Hayman, K., Keeling, S. & Kerse, N. (2009) 'Older people and their social spaces: a study of well-being and attachment to place in Aotearoa New Zealand', *Social Science & Medicine*, vol. 68, pp. 664–671.

Zapf, M. (2009) *Social Work and the Environment: Understanding People and Place*, Canadian Scholars Press, Toronto.

Conclusion: Developing an Agenda to Promote Health and Well-Being in Social Work Education

Beth R. Crisp and Liz Beddoe

To the best of our knowledge, this book (and the journal special issue which preceded it) is the first ever collection of papers on the promotion of health and well-being in social work education inclusive of multiple paradigms. We are pleased that the volume encompasses perspectives on the well-being of students and practitioners as well as the health of service users. It is our hope that this volume will encourage educators and practitioners to incorporate more health content in curriculum and practice. To this extent our aim was to fill a gap that was apparent to us as educators and researchers. Reflecting on their own student experiences, Maidment and Macfarlane have noted that

> ... while notions of illness, oppression and disempowerment were addressed, the notion of 'wellbeing' in a more holistic and creative sense has been widely neglected in traditional social work education. (p. 148)

Similarly, Simpson has commented, well-being as an explicit concept has been absent in the social work literature, or at least in respect of his speciality area of learning disability in the United Kingdom. How typical is the picture painted by Simpson more generally for social workers around the world is unclear, but the chapters in this volume, along with several inquiries from other potential contributors suggest that promoting well-being is of growing concern to many social workers and social work educators.

After we began work on this volume, we found ourselves having conversations in which people assumed that a collection of papers on promoting health and well-being in social work education would be comprised of various considerations of social work responses to the social and emotional aspects of illness and trauma. Whereas historically health social work has been associated with social workers employed in hospitals and health centres, wider understandings of the impact of social environments and access to fundamental resources including adequate housing, education and transport, have enabled a more comprehensive understanding of the role and responsibility of social workers in promoting health and well-being. As Coren et al. have argued:

The key challenge for social workers is to address underlying threats to well-being that may develop into risk. Thus, social work education optimally needs more focus on the interacting factors which contribute to an individual's health, well-being and resources, where there may be no obvious risk of immediate harm but where well-being and quality of life is threatened. (Coren et al., p. 25)

To fully acknowledge the many aspects of human wellbeing—physical, emotional, spiritual, cultural and cognitive—and the link between socioeconomic factors and health inequalities requires social workers to have an understanding of health which goes beyond the biomedical paradigm. In New Zealand and Australia social workers have worked to better understand a holistic approach to health by learning about the spiritual elements so intrinsic to the well-being of indigenous peoples (Durie, 1998; Kaplan-Myrth, 2007). Social work researchers have often sought to avoid narrow paradigms in exploring the well-being of populations served. This is reflected in Beddoe's model curriculum in which students would be taught a series of wide lens and narrow lens questions which they could apply to situations involving a very broad range of health issues. Recognising the impact of culture and environment, Marlowe and Adamson have provided a rationale as to why social workers need a more expansive understanding of trauma than is posited by the International Classification of Diseases (ICD) and Ashcroft charted six influential paradigms which are underpinned by very different understandings of health. In addition, Ashcroft has sought to explain how different perspectives and ways of practising social work result in individual social workers preferring different ways of explaining health. This is important knowledge both for teams of social workers, but just as important for social workers working in interprofessional collaborations as these paradigms can influence how others understand the role of the social worker. Furthermore, as Simpson explains in respect of people with a learning disability, policy responses which have been designed to promote well-being have changed and evolved over recent decades, and at a single point of time there are often substantial geographical variations in approaches.

While it is important that social workers recognize the impact of social determinants on health and well-being and the various paradigms in which health and well-being can be framed, as the remaining chapters in this collection demonstrate, there is a much broader potential for social work education to contribute to the promotion of health and well-being. As Marlowe and Adamson note, this includes the need for a very real rather than superficial understanding of the impact of trauma. An understanding of the positive ways in which migrant, refugee and other populations that are often deemed 'vulnerable' build and sustain community in spite of trauma histories provides us with a deeper appreciation of human resilience. This suggests a necessary reconsideration of the importance of social connectedness (Taket et al., 2009) and for community supports which are outside those staffed by social workers and other health and social care professionals (Crisp, 2010). Social work curricula typically include courses on working in and with human service organisations, which are often busy places, trying to provide quality services despite limited staffing and other resources. Social work theory and practice classes and practice learning may, possibly inadvertently, reinforce a privileging of professional organisations over other community resources in teaching about assessment and referral processes. Although joining craft groups (Maidment and Macfarlane), exploring religious beliefs or participating in religious actions (Crisp) or becoming involved in other community activities such as sporting groups or arts organisations may not be favoured, or even possible, for many service users, as social work educators we nevertheless need to ensure that our students and graduates are able to access and utilise a wide range of community resources and recognise the potential benefits of these resources for community members. Just as importantly, judicious assessment practices need to ensure that our efforts as social workers to provide professional services do not cause further trauma by damaging effective but non-professional community supports.

In addition to promoting health and well-being among the individuals, groups and communities who are served by social workers, a second theme running throughout this volume has been the need to promote the health and well-being of social work students. Napoli and Bonifas remind readers of the immense emotional stresses which are present for many students, some of whom experience their studies as so distressing that they leave before graduation. The case studies of the five final year social work students presented by Hughes explore some of the many tensions and issues which students may face in their quest to qualify, including changing values and outlooks to an extent that this placed strains on relationships which existed prior to commencing study. We also know that those who graduate do not necessarily stay in the profession long-term with a recent British study suggesting that the average working life for a social worker was eight years, compared to 15 for nurses, 25 for doctors and 28 for pharmacists (Curtis et al., 2010). Consequently, in addition to the usual knowledge and skills which are taught to social work students, Napoli and Bonifas, as well as Mensinga have described a range of techniques, including meditation and yoga, which they have used to develop mindfulness in their students. In a profession which values clarity of thought, and indeed several authors in this volume have emphasised the need for expertise in critical thinking, Mensinga, in particular, emphasises the value of workers being aware of the feedback from their own bodies in respect of the stresses they encounter in their work.

A further rationale provided by Napoli and Bonifas for promoting well-being among students is that they will more effectively be able to care for others if they can care for themselves. This may only be possible when expectations on social workers are reasonable and enable them to have an appropriate balance between work and other aspects of their lives. Fouché and Martindale raise the importance of ensuring students understand the importance of maintaining a healthy work–life balance to 'more effectively manage stressors and burnout by addressing the domains that matter most' (p. 17). Developing an understanding of the research underpinning such notions as subjective well-being and work–life balance is of multidimensional significance. The insights gained during social work education will endure to the benefit of students, practitioners and their service users and colleagues alike.

One group whose health and well-being have been virtually ignored in this volume are social work educators, particularly those of us employed in the higher education sector, although Hughes has noted the important role of educators in modelling values and behaviours to social work students. Ironically, many social work educators in our acquaintance work long hours, often far in excess as to what they are paid for in efforts, to be responsive to the complex needs of their students. Perhaps we may pause to ponder whether those emails from students we respond to late at night and at weekends are ultimately helpful if our behaviour models work practices of constant availability and a life of constant work. While we have sometimes laughed at the absurdity of a student emailing or telephoning early on Monday morning to ascertain why their weekend communication to us remains unanswered, the culture in many universities seems to be that working most nights and weekends is an expectation. Stress in the academic workforce is a relevant area for further research (Kinman, 2001). Both of us have been academics for around two decades and are far from alone in experiencing huge increases in workloads, due to student numbers rising at a much faster rate than teaching staff, reductions in administrative support as well as greater expectations on gaining a doctorate, obtaining research grants and publishing books and peer-reviewed articles which can be included in research quality exercises. As senior staff with programme leadership responsibilities including responsibilities for staffing, we have at times been acutely aware of the limitations on us in facilitating reasonable work–life balances not only for ourselves but for colleagues in our programmes.

This is a small collection of chapters and as such cannot reflect all the possible themes and issues apposite to health and well-being in social work education. One of the limitations is that the authors are all from predominantly English-speaking settings in Australia, New Zealand, North America and the United Kingdom. We recognise that the concepts of health and well-being are not universal between cultures and as noted above there is much to be learned from exploring cultural differences in the construction of health and well-being. In Australia and New Zealand, cross-cultural competence, particularly in respect of the indigenous peoples of our countries, is a required skill for social workers and consequently a curriculum requirement in social work education. Some glimpses as to the complexities of cultural competence in respect of health and well-being can be gleaned from Marlowe and Adamson who write about some particular issues for Sudanese refugees in Australia, as well as some Maori viewpoints from New Zealand. In both case studies, the importance of recognising the role of the community when dealing with trauma is considered crucial and is at odds with '"Western" counselling approaches that focussed on talking about trauma in an unfamiliar agency setting' (Marlowe and Adamson, p. 4). Consequently, we can necessarily rely on what were once appropriate methods or processes for promoting health and well-being. As Maidment and Macfarlane have noted:

> ... paradigm shifts in the way people live their lives prompted by the impacts of globalisation necessitate a re-examination of the knowledge base that informs social work and the way it is practiced. The emergence of global ageing, the exponential growth in geographical mobility of kith and kin, rapidly changing technologies and environmental estrangement require practitioners to ... nurture sustainable individual and community wellbeing ... (p. 146)

As have a number of other contributors to this volume, Maidment and Macfarlane suggest that in order to promote well-being, the social work curriculum needs to foster students' abilities to deal with a myriad of complexities which is the lived reality for both individuals and communities. This leads us to question whether as social work educators we need to revisit our definition of social work and to contend that many social workers would be surprised to discover that the enhancement of well-being is so central to the definition of social work adopted by the International Federation of Social Workers in 2000:

> The social work profession promotes social change, problem solving in human relationships and the empowerment and liberation of people to enhance well-being. Utilising theories of human behaviour and social systems, social work intervenes at the points where people interact with their environments. Principles of human rights and social justice are fundamental to social work. (IFSW, 2000)

In reviewing the IFSW definition the Council of Social Work Education Aotearoa New Zealand (Staniforth et al., 2010) links the achievement of well-being with 'positive change'. However, the message which our students receive, either explicitly or implicitly, is that the role of social workers is in the provision of remedial services. For example, in Australia, although the Australian Association of Social Workers (AASW) definition of social work states 'the social work profession is committed to the pursuit of social justice, the enhancement of the quality of life and the development of the full potential of each individual, group and community in society' (AASW, 2010, p. 5), some years ago the association produced a poster, titled 'Social workers make a difference'. The social worker is depicted as constructing a bridge across a deep hole in the ground but despite being built from a wide range of social work skills and practice methods (advocacy, community development, conflict resolution, counselling, crisis work, education, empowerment, family therapy, group work, relationship counselling and social policy) the crossing is incomplete. One possible interpretation of this image is that social workers can put in extensive efforts and even then struggle to ameliorate the difficulties in the lives of service users, let alone improve their well-being. But even when the promotion of well-being is an explicitly stated aim, the impact may be less than optimal if presented as subsequent to social workers meeting other legislative requirements (Scottish Executive, 2003).

There is a challenge for social work educators to question whether the ways in which we define social work may result in students concluding that consideration of health and well-being is an optional extra to some other more pressing or real tasks. Furthermore, we also need to ensure that discussions of health and well-being are not confined to topics concerned with provision of health services. As the IFSW (2008) has noted, all social workers, and not just those employed in the health sector should be playing a role in promoting health and well-being. This may be a greater challenge in countries where the employment of social workers is more narrowly confined to the social services sector (e.g. England and Scotland) than in countries where social workers are employed in a range of sectors, including health services (e.g. Australia, New Zealand, Ireland, North America). However, even when social workers are considered integral to health service provision, the need to conceptualise health issues beyond acute care remains a challenge for social work educators.

Another issue which received very little mention in the papers in this volume, but should increasingly be of concern to social workers is environmental sustainability. The negative impacts on health and well-being due to degradation of air, water and soil disproportionately impact on the poor and marginalised groups in society from whom the users of social work services tend to be associated are starting to be recognised (Berger, 1995; Wiseman, 2007). Energy-efficient heating, cooling and household appliances, solar water heating, installing rainwater tanks, growing fruit and vegetables are among the options which individuals and families may embark upon to both improve their health and well-being and reduce living costs. However, such options may not be possible for those living in rental accommodation or low income home owners, unless they can attract realistic subsidies (KPMG, Brotherhood of St Laurence and Ecos Corporation, 2008). It has been proposed that integrating environmental justice with other social justice issues should be a key challenge for social work, although it is recognised that how social workers incorporate such thinking into their work will require a re-thinking about how social work is understood and practiced (Zapf, 2009).

Finally, we need to ensure that the process of social work education promotes the health and well-being of both social work students and those who teach them. While there is plenty of justification that prospective social workers be able to demonstrate a high degree of competence in responding to complex social problems, we nevertheless need to ensure that the demands on either students or ourselves are not unduly onerous (Crisp et al., 2003). Furthermore, we need to ensure that the skills and knowledge which promote professional resilience are considered no less integral in social work education than the skills and knowledge to effectively promote the health and well-being of the individuals, families and communities which social workers are charged to work with. There is ample evidence in the literature to describe social workers' jobs as being stressful in nature and for stress to impact on well-being (Collins, 2007, 2008; DePanfilis, 2006). Negative workplace experiences are thought to contribute to ongoing recruitment and retention challenges faced by the profession as workers leave their jobs for roles that they perceive to be less emotionally demanding (DePanfilis, 2006). High turnover has a deleterious effect on all the stakeholders of a social service organisation, from service users and carers, to managers and practitioners and this may perpetuate the cycle of difficulty found in this context in the first instance. We do not wish to unduly emphasise the profession as being inherently 'stressful'; indeed there is an extensive body of research emerging which supports the view that, despite working in often adverse conditions, social workers experience high levels of job satisfaction (Collins, 2008). Congruently, resiliency frameworks advance a strengths-based approach to this issue and focus on identifying variables that underpin subjective well-being (Graham & Shier, 2010) so that alternative strategies can emerge to support the development of resiliency in social workers, especially during social work education (Beddoe, Davys & Adamson, 2011; Grant & Kinman, 2012).

There are clearly many challenges for the profession of social work and for social work educators in particular, in promoting health and well-being, and this volume only begins to explore these issues. Nevertheless, sometimes it seems as if sections of the profession do not share our view that the promotion of health and well-being is a fundamental aim of social work, and perhaps overcoming this is the greatest challenge we face as educators.

References

Australian Association of Social Workers (AASW) (2010) *Australian Social Work Education and Accreditation Standards, 2010*. Canberra, AASW.

Beddoe, L., Davys, A., & Adamson, C. (2011) 'Educating resilient practitioners', *Social Work Education*. doi:10.1080/02615479.2011.644532

Berger, R. M. (1995) 'Habitat destruction syndrome', *Social Work*, vol. 40, no. 4, pp. 441–443.

Collins, S. (2007) 'Social workers, resilience, positive emotions and optimism', *Practice*, vol. 19, no. 4, pp. 255–269.

Collins, S. (2008) 'Statutory social workers: Stress, job satisfaction, coping, social support and individual differences', *British Journal of Social Work*, vol. 38, no. 6, pp. 1173–1193.

Crisp, B. R. (2010) *Spirituality and Social Work*, Ashgate, Farnham.

Crisp, B. R., Anderson, M. R., Orme, J. & Green Lister, P. (2003) *Knowledge Review 1: Learning and Teaching in Social Work Education—Assessment*, Policy Press, Bristol.

Curtis, L., Moriarty, J. & Netten, A. (2010) 'The expected working life of a social worker', *British Journal of Social Work*, vol. 40, no. 5, pp. 1628–1643.

DePanfilis, D. (2006) 'Compassion fatigue, burnout, and compassion satisfaction: Implications for retention of workers', *Child Abuse & Neglect*, vol. 30, no. 10, pp. 1067–1069.

Durie, M. (1998) *Whaiora: Maori health development*, 2nd edition, Oxford University Press, Auckland.

Graham, J. & Shier, M. L. (2010) 'Social work practitioners and subjective well-being: Personal factors that contribute to high levels of subjective well-being', *International Social Work*, vol. 53, no. 6, pp. 757–772.

Grant, L. & Kinman, G. (2012) 'Enhancing wellbeing in social work students: Building resilience in the next generation', *Social Work Education*. vol. 31, no. 5, pp. 605–621.

International Federation of Social Workers (IFSW) (2000) *Definition of Social Work*. Available at http://www.ifsw.org/f38000138.html, accessed 2 January 2012.

International Federation of Social Workers (IFSW) (2008) *International Policy on Health*. Available at http://www.ifsw.org/en/p38000081.html, accessed 30 November 2011.

Kaplan-Myrth, N. (2007) *Hard Yakka: Transforming Indigenous Health Policy and Politics*, Lexington Books, Lanham, MD.

Kinman, G. (2001) 'Pressure Points: A review of research on stressors and strains in UK academics', *Educational Psychology*, vol. 21, no. 4, pp. 473–492.

KPMG, Brotherhood of St Laurence and Ecos Corporation (2008) A National Energy Efficiency Program to Assist Low-income Households. Australia, KPMG. Available at http://www.bsl.org.au/pdfs/KPMG_national_energy_efficiency_program_low-income_households.pdf, accessed 2 January 2012.

Scottish Executive (2003) *The Framework for Social Work Education in Scotland*, The Stationery Office, Edinburgh.

Staniforth, B., Beddoe, L. & Henrickson, M. (2010) *Report from CSWEANZ Social Work Definition Workshop*, Auckland University 3 December 2010, Council of Social Work Education Aotearoa New Zealand.

Taket, A., Crisp, B.R., Nevill, A., Lamaro, G., Graham, M. & Barter-Godfrey, S. (eds) (2009) *Theorising Social Exclusion*, Routledge, Abingdon.

Wiseman, J. (2007) 'Climate change and social justice: Towards an Australian research and policy agenda', *Just Policy*, no. 46, pp. 8–11.

Zapf, M. (2009) *Social Work and the Environment: Understanding People and Place*, Canadian Scholars' Press, Toronto.